Diabetes

Chronic Complications

Diabetes

Chronic Complications

Editors

Kenneth M. Shaw and Michael H. Cummings

Queen Alexandra Hospital, Portsmouth, UK

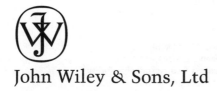

John Wiley & Sons, Ltd

Copyright © 2005   John Wiley & Sons Ltd, The Atrium, Southern Gate, Chichester,
West Sussex PO19 8SQ, England

Telephone   (+44) 1243 779777

Email (for orders and customer service enquiries): cs-books@wiley.co.uk
Visit our Home Page on www.wileyeurope.com or www.wiley.com

Reprinted with corrections February 2006

Other Wiley Editorial Offices

John Wiley & Sons Inc., 111 River Street, Hoboken, NJ 07030, USA

Jossey-Bass, 989 Market Street, San Francisco, CA 94103-1741, USA

Wiley-VCH Verlag GmbH, Boschstr. 12, D-69469 Weinheim, Germany

John Wiley & Sons Australia Ltd, 42 McDougall Street, Milton, Queensland 4064, Australia

John Wiley & Sons (Asia) Pte Ltd, 2 Clementi Loop #02-01, Jin Xing Distripark, Singapore 129809

John Wiley & Sons Canada Ltd, 22 Worcester Road, Etobicoke, Ontario, Canada M9W 1L1

Wiley also publishes its books in a variety of electronic formats. Some content that appears in print may not
be available in electronic books.

Library of Congress Cataloging-in-Publication Data

Diabetes : chronic complications / editors, Kenneth M. Shaw and Michael H. Cummings. – 2nd ed.
        p.; cm.
    Rev. ed. of: Diabetic complications / edited by K.M. Shaw. c1996.
    Includes bibliographical references and index.
    ISBN-13 978-0-470-86579-8
    ISBN-10 0-470-86579-2
    1. Diabetes–Complications.   I. Shaw, K. (Kenneth)   II. Cummings, Michael H.
        III. Diabetic Complications.
    [DNLM: 1. Diabetes Complications.   WK 835 D5343 2005]
    RC660.D5636 2005
    616. 4'62–dc22   2005019919

British Library Cataloguing in Publication Data

A catalogue record for this book is available from the British Library
ISBN-13 978-0-470-86579-8 (P/B)
ISBN-10 0-470-86579-2 (P/B)

Typeset in 10.5/13pt Times by Thomson Press (India) Limited, New Delhi
Printed and bound in Great Britain by Antony Rowe, Chippenham, Wilts
This book is printed on acid-free paper responsibly manufactured from sustainable forestry
in which at least two trees are planted for each one used for paper production.

Contents

Preface to *Diabetic Complications*

We appear to be on the threshold of witnessing a substantial reduction in the long-term complications of diabetes. Modern treatment regimens, better monitoring of control and the huge impact of improved education all combine to offer the prospect of real progress towards prevention of complications and lessening of progression in those in whom complications may be present. The Diabetes Control and Complications Trial (DCCT) has provided eveidence that such can be achieved, while the St Vincent Declaration initiative has set the standards to enable these benefits to become reality. Such is the encouraging future expectation that the logistics of delivering the necessary diabetes care to achieve the potential immense health gain are still daunting. Much more diabetes care is being undertaken in general practice as structured mini-clinics are established, while hospital diabetes centres have never been busier as more specialized complex cases are referred. Never has organized multiprofessional teamwork across all sectors of health care been needed more. Whether the patient is managed at a hospital centre, in a community mini-clinic or on a shared-care basis, the importance of identifying those patients at risk of complications and the detection of developing complications at an early stage is now beyond dispute.

The contributors to this book have extensive experience in diabetes, either as specialists specifically in diabetes or as experts in other fields to whom complications of diabetes are referred. Each contribution seeks to outline the nature of diabetes complications, how susceptibility and risk can be identified, the importance of screening during the early stages and the way appropriate investigation and management should be undertaken.

It is hoped that those of all disciplines involved in the day-to-day care and education of diabetes, either in the community or in the specialist centre, will find both interest and practical help from the content of this book. The St Vincent's objective of reducing and even eliminating complications of diabetes is now a real and achievable goal.

K.M. SHAW
Portsmouth, February 1996

Foreword to *Diabetic Complications*

Nearly three-quarters of a century has passed since the discovery of insulin, and while there is scarcely anyone who can now recall diabetes treatment before 1922, there are many whose memories extend over 60 years or more to the early exhilarating era of insulin treatment. Some recall their physicians of the time, notably perhaps Dr. R. D. Lawrence of King's College Hospital, that flamboyant, yet astute and most caring of physicians. Yet those with long memories and long lives have survived a life of diabetes, happily spared the development of diabetic complications. The absence of complications may have been due in part to good management, but a genetic influence is probably as important.

The euphoria of the 1920s was followed by recognition of most of the disorders due to diabetic complications in the following decades. Yet by mid-century physicians could only observe the outcome with little change of having any influence on the natural progression of the disease. Nephropathy and retinopathy frequently led to renal failure and blindness, while the consequences of neuropathy and vascular disease resulted in catastrophic foot disease and amputations.

In the last 25 years there has been a dramatic change. The benefits of tight metabolic control have been demonstrated in numerous studies, most recently and most conclusively in the Diabetes Control arid Complications Trial (DCCT) in the USA. It is now possible to reduce the incidence of complications by 35–70 per cent, or when they occur to retard their progression. This magnificent study gives enormous encouragement to both patients and their physicians and nurses by demonstrating that their efforts are really worthwhile. It gives renewed impetus to the search for achieving better diabetes control without developing the devastating consequences of hypoglycaemia.

Extraordinary developments have also evolved in treating the consequences of diabetic complications when they do occur. In Germany, photocoagulation was used empirically to prevent the evolution of retinopathy and was subsequently shown to prevent blindness. The evolution of nephropathy can be substantially reduced by hypotensive treatment, and the potential specific advantage of angiotensin-converting enzyme inhibitors has been demonstrated. Dialysis and transplantation are now available to most diabetic patients who need renal support treatment, although even a decade ago, many centres considered that diabetic patients did not qualify for these treatments. The availability especially of continuous ambulatory peritoneal dialysis (CAPD) has transformed the availability of renal support even in elderly patients who can achieve a very acceptable quality of life. Treatment of the diabetic foot has been revolutionized: primary prevention of foot ulcers by education, chiropody and advice on footwear represents probably the best and most cost-effective prevention measure in the care of diabetic patients. The establishment of specialized foot clinics leads to rapid treatment of threatening lesions, and the amputation rate can thereby be halved. Angioplasty and vascular surgery have advanced to the point where they make an important contribution to limb salvage.

Proper care in the 1990s must therefore include the facilities for identification of all patients with diabetes – hence the need for diabetes registers – and regular review for early detection of complications, which will enable physicians to take the steps needed to abort the disease. These requirements place a huge demand on society in terms of health resources, but the demands of our patients are now heard, and governments have acknowledged the need to reduce complications following wide acceptance of the St Vincent declarations. So it is the organization of diabetes care which must change to accommodate these developments. The introduction of the diabetes specialist nurse is probably the most important innovation is diabetes care, and his/her expertise now enables delivery of care on a community basis, linked of course to the strength of diabetes expertise and research at the hospital-based diabetes departments. These new arrangements must be made to achieve high standards, and there should be a new era of optimism which might lead to a reduction of the tragedies of diabetes, just as improved standards reduced foetal mortality from over 30 per cent in the 1940s to between 1 and 2 per cent in the 1990s.

This book addresses these topical issues in a comprehensive approach, and describes in detail methods for early detection of diabetes complications by the extended team ranging from the community base to the hospital. Specialist nurses are responsible for one of the chapters, giving an indication of their key role not just in the care of patients, but also in the organization of screening and education programmes, now crucial to the provision of high-quality diabetes care.

There can be few fields in medicine in which such important advances have been made in little more than two decades. As the British Diabetic Association, which has done so much to advance understanding of the disease and help public understanding of its needs, celebrates its 60th birthday, both those with diabetes and those who care for them should have a renewed optimism for the future. The advances stem, of course, from the events in 1922 when the earliest patients were treated with C insulin, and Elizabeth Hughes wrote to her mother that 'Dr Banting considers my progress simply miraculous'. The advances continue to this day.

P. J. WATKINS
Diabetic Department
King's College Hospital, London

Preface to the Current Edition

The exponential rise in the global prevalence of diabetes, particularly type 2, but also type 1 at young age, will almost certainly be associated with an inevitable and parallel increase in the long-term complications that associate with diabetes. Both metabolic susceptibility and complication predisposition are subject to genetic determination, but the expression of such is significantly influenced by environmental factors. The substantial rise in numbers with diabetes would indicate that adverse lifestyle factors continue largely unabated and, despite advances in understanding and therapy, consequent complications are set to continue, albeit with changing patterns.

The long-term complications of diabetes are well known and such is the diversity of effect that new areas of adverse consequence continue to be identified, such as non-alcoholic fatty liver disease, increased risk of colorectal cancer with insulin-resistance and psychological disturbance such as depression. Furthermore, diabetes is a great magnifier and so often physical ailments are worsened by diabetes if not directly caused by it.

Yet, an increasing evidence base provides encouragement that the development of diabetic complications can at least be ameliorated if not prevented. DCCT for type 1 and UK PDS for type 2 diabetes have shown that for microangiopathy a reduction in complication rate can be achieved and furthermore the benefit continues even when intensive management is lessened. On the other hand, for large vessel disease, although the relationship of hyperglycaemia to causation is established, so far the benefits of improved glycaemic control are uncertain. In this context, other vascular risk factors are seemingly more important.

The pattern of diabetic complications is changing. In Western Europe advanced retinal disease and end stage renal failure are diminishing, whilst coronary heart disease has become the greatest clinical challenge. This change will have resulted from a number of advances in clinical management – better screening, better therapies and better monitoring – but there is still much more to be done to reduce the considerable burden of diabetic complications on the individual and society. Present therapeutic strategies are predominantly based on surrogate indicators of risk, and hence tend to be target-driven. Whether such intensified strategies will prove effective remains to be seen. Meanwhile, education and understanding promoting healthier lifestyles remain paramount.

Since the first edition of *Diabetes: Chronic Complications*, many advances have been made. Once more for this new edition we have drawn upon contributors with extensive experience in diabetes or specialist experience of issues related to diabetes. Again we have endeavoured to ensure that, along with an understanding of the nature of diabetic complications, a clear and practical guidance is provided on appropriate management. The evidence base for the reduction of diabetic complications is positive and encouraging, but the achievement of successful outcomes is still less easily implemented in this world of increasing diabetes. This second edition sets out to provide for all those involved in diabetes care a greater awareness of the problems encountered along with pragmatic advice on practice management.

KENNETH M. SHAW
MICHAEL H. CUMMINGS
Queen Alexandra Hospital
Portsmouth

List of Contributors

Duncan L. Browne Consultant Physician in Diabetes and Endocrinology, Royal Cornwall Hospitals. Truro, Cornwall

Angela Cook Humming Bird Centre, Royal Shrewsbury Hospital, Shrewsbury, SY3 8XQ, UK

Iain Cranston Queen Alexandra Hospital, Cosham, Portsmouth, Hampshire PO6 3LY, UK

Michael H. Cummings Academic Department of Diabetes and Endocrinology, Queen Alexandra Hospital, Southwick Hill Road, Cosham, Portsmouth, Hampshire PO6 3LY, UK

Grant Duncan Queen Mary's Hospital, Roehampton, London SW15 5PN, UK

Anton V. Emmanuel Physiology Unit, St Marks Hospital, Watford Road, Harrow HA1 3UJ, UK

Miles Fisher Royal Alexandra Hospital, Corsebar Road, Paisley, Strathclyde PA2 9PN, UK

Adam Haworth Department of Dermatology, St Mary's Hospital, Milton Road, Portsmouth PO3 6AD, UK

Emma Holland Queen Alexandra Hospital, Cosham, Portsmouth, Hampshire PO6 3LY, UK

Deborah Land Portsmouth Hospitals NHS Trust, Portsmouth, UK

Richard MacIsaac Endocrinology Unit, Austin Health, University of Melbourne, Heidelberg, Victoria 3084, Australia

Andrew Macleod Royal Shrewsbury Hospital, Mytton Oak Road, Shrewsbury SY3 8XQ, UK

Fiona C. McCrae Rheumatology Department, Queen Alexandra Hospital, Cosham, Portsmouth, Hampshire PO6, UK

Darryl Meeking Queen Alexandra Hospital, Cosham, Portsmouth, Hampshire, PO6 3LY, UK

Charles D. R. Murray   Physiology Unit, St Marks Hospital, Watford Road, Harrow HA1 3UJ, UK

Kenneth M. Shaw   Queen Alexandra Hospital, Cosham, Portsmouth, Hampshire PO6 3LY, UK

Kevin Shotliff   Queen Mary's Hospital, Roehampton, London SW15 5PN, UK

Gerald Watts   Department of Medicine, The University of Western Australia, PO X2213, GPO, Perth, Australia

1

Diabetes and the Eye

Kevin Shotliff and **Grant Duncan**

1.1   Introduction

Since the invention of the direct ophthalmoscope by Helmholtz in 1851 and
von Yaeger's first description of changes in the fundus of a person with diabetes
4 years later, there has been increasing interest in the retina as it contains the only
part of the vasculature affected by diabetes that is easily visible. Interestingly, these
first retinal changes described in 1855 were actually hypertensive, not diabetic.

Despite the target outlined in the St Vincent Declaration in 1989 to reduce
blindness caused by diabetes by one-third within 5 years, and the advances made
in laser therapy and vitreoretinal surgical techniques, diabetic retinopathy remains
the commonest cause of blindness in the working-age population of the Western
world. Furthermore, with predictions of a dramatic increase in the number of
people diagnosed with diabetes, the detection and treatment of diabetic retinopathy
continues to be a focal point for healthcare professionals. Indeed the recent
National Service Framework for Diabetes (NSF) has prioritized diabetic retinopathy by setting specific targets associated with retinal screening and implement-
ing the development of a National Screening Programme.

Visual loss from diabetic retinopathy has two main causes: maculopathy,
described as disruption of the macular region of the retina, leading to impairment
of central vision; and retinal ischaemia, resulting in proliferative diabetic retinopathy.

As well as the retina, other parts of the eye can also be affected in people with
diabetes. Cataracts are more prevalent and are actually the most common eye
abnormality seen in people with diabetes, occurring in up to 60 per cent of 30–
54-year-olds. The link between diabetes and primary open angle glaucoma,
however, continues to be disputed. Vitreous changes do occur in people with

Diabetes: Chronic Complications   Edited by Kenneth M. Shaw and Michael H. Cummings
© 2005 John Wiley & Sons, Ltd.

diabetes, such as asteroid hyalosis, seen in about 2 per cent of patients. These small spheres or star-shaped opacities in the vitreous appear to sparkle when illuminated and do not normally affect vision. Branch retinal vein occlusions and central retinal vein occlusions are associated with hypertension, hyperlipidaemia and obesity, and are often found in people with diabetes. Hypertensive retinopathy features several lesions in common with diabetic retinopathy, and care must be taken not to confuse the two conditions.

1.2   Epidemiology of Diabetic Retinopathy

Currently 2 per cent of the UK diabetic population is thought to be registered blind,[1] which means that a person with diabetes has a 10- to 20-fold increased risk of blindness. The prevalence of diabetic retinopathy depends on multiple factors and, like many microvascular complications, is more common in the ethnic minorities compared with Caucasians.

A prevalence of 25–30 per cent for a general diabetic population is often quoted. Every year about one in 90 North Americans with diabetes develops proliferative retinopathy and one in 80 develops macula oedema.

In type 1 patients:[2,3]

- <2 per cent have any lesions of diabetic retinopathy at diagnosis;

- 8 per cent have it by 5 years (2 per cent proliferative);

- 87–98 per cent have abnormalities 30 years later (30 per cent of these having had proliferative retinopathy).

In type 2 patients:[4,5]

- 20–37 per cent can be expected to have retinopathy at diagnosis;

- 15 years later, 85 per cent of those on insulin and 60 per cent of those on diet or oral agents will have abnormalities.

The 4-year incidence of proliferative retinopathy in a large North American epidemiological study was 10.5 per cent in type 1 patients, 7.4 per cent in older onset/type 2 patients taking insulin and 2.3 per cent in type 2 patients not on insulin.[2,3,5]

Currently in the UK, maculopathy is a more common and therefore more significant sight-threatening complication of diabetes. This is due to the much greater number of people with type 2 diabetes compared with type 1 and the fact that maculopathy tends to occur in older people. About 75 per cent of those with maculopathy have type 2 diabetes and there is a 4-year incidence of 10.4 per cent in this group.[5] Although type 2 patients are 10 times more likely to have maculopathy than type 1 patients, 14 per cent of type 1 patients who become blind do so because of maculopathy.[1]

The risk factors for development/worsening of diabetic retinopathy are:

- duration of diabetes;

- type of diabetes (proliferative disease in type 1 and maculopathy in type 2);

- poor diabetic/glycaemic control;

- hypertension;

- diabetic nephropathy;

- recent cataract surgery;

- pregnancy;

- alcohol (variable results which may be related to the type of alcohol involved, e.g. effects are worse in Scotland than in Italy);

- smoking (variable results, but appears worse in young people with exudates and older women with proliferative disease);

- ethnic origin.

1.3 Retinal Anatomy

To understand how diabetic retinopathy is classified and treated, a basic grasp of retinal anatomy is essential. The retina is the innermost of three successive layers of the globe of the eye, the others being:

- the sclera–the rigid outer covering of the eye, which includes the cornea;

- the choroid–the highly vascularized middle layer of the eye, which has the largest blood flow in the entire body.

The retina comprises two parts: the pars optica retinae, the photoreceptive part composed of nine layers; and the pars caeca retinae, a non-receptive part forming the pigment epithelium (Figure 1.1).

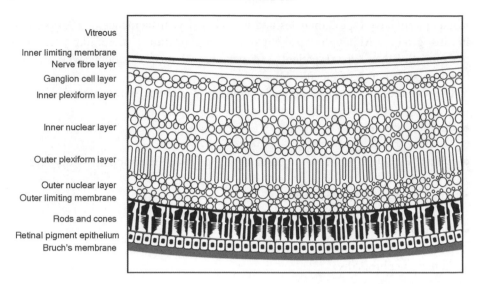

Vitreous
Inner limiting membrane
Nerve fibre layer
Ganglion cell layer
Inner plexiform layer
Inner nuclear layer
Outer plexiform layer
Outer nuclear layer
Outer limiting membrane
Rods and cones
Retinal pigment epithelium
Bruch's membrane

Figure 1.1 Cross-section of the retina illustrating the 10 layers of the retina: inner limiting membrane (glial cell fibres forming the barrier between the retina and the vitreous body), optic nerve fibres (axons of the third neuron), ganglion cells (cell nuclei of multipolar ganglion cells of the third neuron), inner plexiform layer (synapses between axons of the second neuron and dendrites of the third neuron), inner nuclear layer (cell nuclei of the bipolar nerve cells of the second neuron), outer plexiform layer (synapses between axons of the first neuron and dendrites of the second neuron), outer nuclear layer (cell nuclei of rods and cones, the first neuron), outer limiting membrane (porous plate of processes of glial cells, which rods and cones project through), rods and cones (true photoreceptors), retinal pigment epithelium (single layer of pigmented epithelial cells) and Bruch's membrane

The normal retina is completely transparent, its bright red/orange reflex the result of the underlying vasculature of the choroid. The retina has a number of distinct features. The optic nerve (often described as the optic disc) is a circular structure varying in colour from pale pink in the young to yellow/orange in older people. It is located approximately 15° nasally from the visual axis and slightly superior (Figure 1.2). The optic nerve is essentially a 'cable' connecting the eye to the brain, which carries information from the retina to the visual cortex via the optic chiasm. The optic nerve may exhibit a central depression known as the optic or physiologic cup. Both the central retinal vein and artery leave and enter the eye through the optic nerve. The 'blind spot' on visual field testing occurs because the optic disc contains no photoreceptor rod and cone cells.

The macula is the round area at the posterior pole within the temporal vessel arcades 3–4 mm temporal to and slightly lower than the optic disc (Figure 1.2). It is approximately 5 mm in diameter. At the centre of the macula and roughly the same size as the optic disc is the fovea, a depression in the retinal surface. The fovea is the point at which vision is sharpest; the foveola, the thinnest part of the retina and forming the base of the fovea, contains only cone cells, giving this

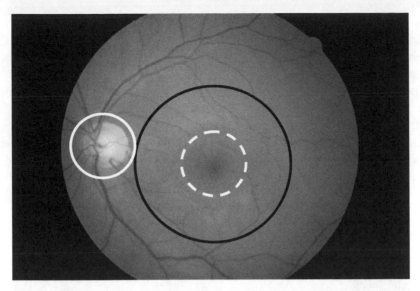

Figure 1.2 Fundus photograph illustrating the normal retina with optic nerve head (optic disc) circled in white, macula circled in black and the fovea circled with a broken white line

area such well-defined vision. At the very centre of the foveola lies the umbo, a tiny depression corresponding to the foveolar reflex.

The fovea features an avascular zone of variable diameter extending beyond the foveola (Figure 1.3).

The five innermost layers of the retina, from the inner limiting membrane to inner nuclear layer receive their blood supply from the central artery of the retina.

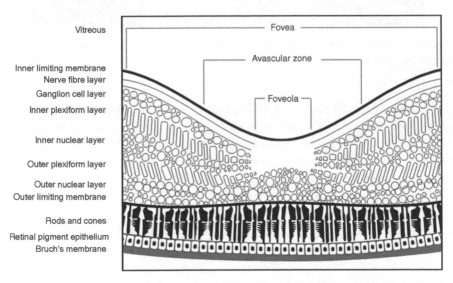

Figure 1.3 Cross-section of the retina at the fovea illustrating the fovea, the foveola and the foveal avascular zone

This enters the retina at the optic disc and forms four branches. The five outer layers of the retina, from the outer plexiform layer to the pigment epithelium, receive their blood supply from the capillaries of the choroid by means of diffusion.

The retinal veins exit the retina at the optic disc and with the arteries form the four vessel arcades of the retina–superior and inferior temporal arcades and superior and inferior nasal arcades (Figure 1.4). Retinal arteries appear bright red, with a sharp reflex strip which becomes lighter with age, and retinal veins are a darker red with little or no reflex strip.

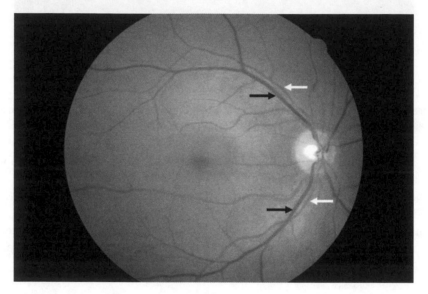

Figure 1.4   Retinal veins (black arrows) and retinal arteries (white arrows) of the superior and inferior temporal arcades

The retinal pigment epithelium (RPE) is the base layer of the retina. The level of adhesion between the RPE and the sensory retina is weaker than that between the RPE and Bruch's membrane, resulting in a potential space. A retinal detachment is the separation of the sensory retina from the RPE as a result of subretinal fluid infiltrating this potential space.

1.4   Classification/Clinical and Histological Features of Diabetic Retinopathy

The classification of diabetic retinopathy as shown in Figure 1.5 is based on visible/ophthalmoscopic features, but unseen changes occurring before these help

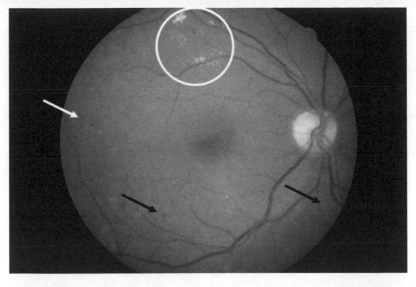

Figure 1.5 Background diabetic retinopathy with microaneurysm (white arrow), haemorrhages (black arrows) and hard exudates (white circles)

explain the clinical findings. Amongst the first are thickening of the capillary basement membrane and loss of the pericytes embedded in it.

As the basement membrane thickens, it loses its negative charge and becomes 'leakier'. In normal retinal capillaries there is a 1:1 relationship between endothelial cells and pericytes, which is the highest ratio for any capillary network in the body. Pericytes may control endothelial cell proliferation, maintain the structural integrity of capillaries and regulate blood flow. This along with increased blood viscosity, abnormal fibrinolytic activity and reduced red cell deformity may lead to capillary occlusion, tissue hypoxia and the stimulus for new vessel formation.

While the toxicity of glucose/hyperglycaemia is accepted, exactly how locally produced growth factors, altered protein kinase C activity, alterations in oxidative stress responses and alterations in the autoregulation of retinal blood flow combine to cause this remains unclear, but is avidly debated.

The natural progression is from background to pre-proliferative/pre-maculopathy then to proliferative retinopathy/maculopathy and ultimately sight-threatening disease.

Background retinopathy (Figure 1.5)

- Capillary microaneurysms are the earliest feature seen clinically, as red 'dots'.

- Small intraretinal haemorrhages or 'blots' also occur, as can haemorrhage into the nerve fibre layer, often flame-shaped.

- With increased capillary leakage hard exudates, lipid deposits, also occur.

Pre-proliferative retinopathy (Figure 1.6)

- Cotton wool spots or soft exudates are infarcts in the nerve fibre layer which alter axoplasmic transport in ganglion cell neurones, giving oedematous infarcts that are seen as pale/grey fuzzy-edged lesions.

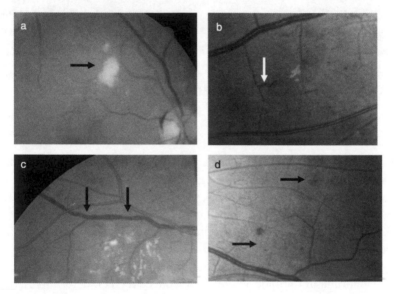

Figure 1.6   Pre-proliferative diabetic retinopathy with (a) cotton wool spots, (b) venous loop, (c) venous beading and (d) IRMA

- Intra-retinal microvascular abnormalities (IRMAs) are tortuous dilated hyper-cellular capillaries in the retina, which enlarge enough to be visible and occur in response to retinal ischaemia.

- Further changes include alternating dilatation and constriction of veins (venous beading) and other venous alterations such as duplication and loop formation.

- There are also large areas of capillary non-perfusion occurring in the absence of new vessels. These ischaemic areas may not be visible with an ophthalmoscope but can be seen on fluorescein angiography.

The Early Treatment of Diabetic Retinopathy Study (ETDRS) suggested that certain of these features matter and suggested a '4–2–1' rule:[6]

- four quadrants of severe haemorrhages or microaneurysms;

- two quadrants of IRMAs;

- one quadrant with venous beading.

If a patient has one of these features, there is a 15 per cent risk of developing sight-threatening retinopathy within the next year. If two are present this rises to a 45 per cent risk.

Proliferative retinopathy (Figure 1.7)

New vessels form and grow along, into or out from the retina. A scaffolding for fibrosis then forms. There are two forms of new vessels:

- those on the disc or within one disc diameter of the disc (NVD);

- new vessels elsewhere (NVE).

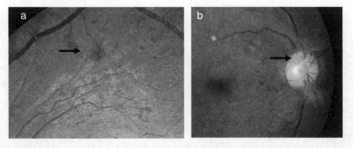

Figure 1.7 Proliferative diabetic retinopathy with (a) neovascularization on the surface of the retina (NVE) and (b) neovascularization at the optic disc (NVD)

Both give no symptoms but cause the problems of advanced retinopathy (Figure 1.8) such as haemorrhage, scar tissue formation, traction on the retina and retinal detachment, which actually results in loss of vision. That is why pan-retinal photocoagulation, which can result in the regression of these new vessels, is used when they are seen.

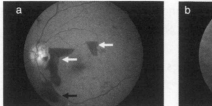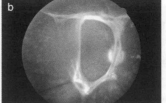

Figure 1.8 Advanced diabetic retinopathy with (a) pre-retinal haemorrhages (white arrows) and vitreous haemorrhage (black arrow) and (b) fibrous proliferation

Diabetic maculopathy

Oedema in the macula area can distort central vision and reduce visual acuity. Any of the above changes can co-exist with maculopathy. The changes seen can be:

- oedematous (clinically it may just be difficult to focus on the macula with a hand-held ophthalmoscope, or visual acuity may have altered or may worsen when a pin hole is used);

- exudative (with haemorrhages, hard exudates and circinate exudates; Figure 1.9);

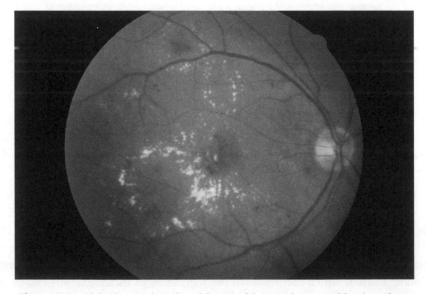

Figure 1.9 Diabetic maculopathy with retinal haemorrhages and hard exudates

- ischaemic (capillary loss occurs but clinically the macula may look normal on direct ophthalmoscopy, although poorly perfused areas will show up on fluorescein angiography);

- Any combination of these (Figure 1.10).

Background retinopathy (grade R1)

- Microaneurysms
- Haemorrhages
- Hard exudates

Preproliferative retinopathy (grade R2)

- Soft exudates/cotton wool spots
- Intra-retinal microvascular abnormalities (IRMAs)
- Venous abnormalities (e.g. venous beading, looping and reduplication)

Proliferative retinopathy (grade R3)

- New vessels on the disc or within 1 disc diameter of it (NVD)
- New vessels elsewhere (NVE)
- Rubeosis iridis ($\pm$ neovascular glaucoma)

Maculopathy (grade M)

- Haemorrhages and hard exudates in the macula area
- Reduced visual acuity with no abnormality seen

Other Grades:

R0: Normal fundus appearance
A: Advanced eye disease including vitreous haemorrhage, fibrosis and retinal detachments
P: Evidence of previous laser therapy
U: Un-gradable image
OL: Other non-diabetic changes/lesion seen

Figure 1.10 Classification, features and grading scheme for diabetic retinopathy

Eye screening

Diabetic retinopathy meets the World Health Organization's four cardinal principles which determine whether a health problem is suitable for screening. These are:

(1) The condition should be an important health problem with a recognizable pre-symptomatic state – as the commonest cause of blindness in the working population of the Western world with a well-recognized pattern of changes visible in the eye, diabetic retinopathy fulfills this.

(2) An appropriate screening procedure, which is acceptable both to the public and health care professionals, should be available – retinal photography is accepted by patients and the medical profession.

(3) Treatment for patients with recognizable disease should be safe, effective and universally agreed – laser therapy for advanced disease, although not without risk, is accepted as a good evidence-based therapy to prevent blindness, and newer medical therapies are in development.

(4) The economic cost of early diagnosis and treatment should be considered in relation to total expenditure on health care, including the consequences of leaving the disease untreated.

To detect diabetic retinopathy the retina must first be visualized. Several methods of retinal examination can be used:

- Indirect ophthalmoscopy with a slit lamp bio-microscope performed by an ophthalmologist is considered to be the gold standard for diagnosing diabetic retinopathy.

- The direct method, using a hand-held ophthalmoscope is performed as part of everyday practice by many doctors. The practicalities of ophthalmoscopy, including the high costs in terms of the level of specialist training and experience required (indirect method), varying results depending on the person carrying out the examination (direct method) and the fact that no permanent visual record is retained (both methods), mean that ophthalmoscopy has been deemed unsuitable as the basis for a comprehensive national screening programme.[7]

- Digital retinal photography (Figure 1.11) with mydriasis provides a permanent record, which can be interpreted with a high degree of accuracy and is relatively inexpensive. Photography and grading of resulting images by trained technicians have demonstrated a higher level of sensitivity and specificity than any other screening method and provide a permanent record for quality assurance and audit.

In light of this, the National Screening Committee has therefore recommended digital retinal photography as the screening method of choice.[8] A comprehensive national screening programme is currently being implemented to meet targets set out in the National Service Framework (NSF) for diabetes. Although NSF targets are based on annual screening, results from a study by the Royal Liverpool University Hospital concluded that a 3 year screening interval may be appropriate for patients with no retinopathy and well-controlled diabetes.[9] During pregnancy,

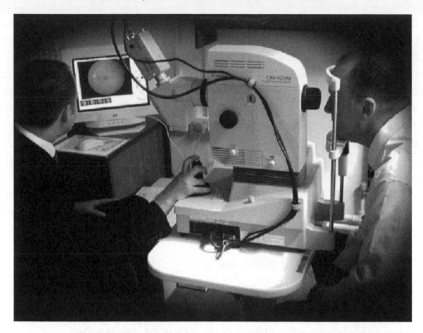

Figure 1.11 Screening for diabetic retinopathy using a digital fundus camera

women with diabetes should be screened each trimester, regardless of their level of control or the absence of any existing retinopathy.

A full retinal screening examination should include:

(1) Visual acuity (VA) – using a standard Snellen Chart; if VA is worse than 6/9 it should be rechecked with a pinhole to correct for refractive errors. If it does not then correct to 6/9 or better, or if it has worsened by more than two lines on a Snellen chart in the last year, an ophthalmology review may be needed as some maculopathy cannot be seen easily with a hand-held ophthalmoscope. Cataracts are, however, a more likely cause. If vision gets worse with a pinhole, it should be assumed that maculopathy is there until proven otherwise. It should be remembered that high blood glucose readings can give myopia (difficulty in distance vision) and low blood glucose hypermetropia (difficulty in reading), although this is not universal.

(2) Examination of the eye through a dilated pupil – although retinal photography has overtaken this, the ability to examine an eye, including the anterior chamber, lens and fundus, should not be lost as a skill, since significant disease is often picked up using this method in opportunistic screening and in those who cannot get to a site where photography is possible, such as the bed-bound and infirm in nursing homes.

(3) Retinal photographs – over 90 per cent of people can have good quality photographs performed. Historically this used Polaroid film, then 35 mm slide film. Now digital images are used as they require a less intense flash and can be repeated immediately if the view is inadequate. The photographs/images obtained should then be graded/assessed by a trained observer using a standardized grading scheme, as demonstrated in Figure 1.10. In the future, scanning laser ophthalmoscopes and computer grading software may also be used.

Reasons for immediate referral to an ophthalmologist are:

• proliferative retinopathy – untreated NVD carries a 40 per cent risk of blindness in under 2 years and laser treatment reduces this;

• rubeosis iridis/neovascular glaucoma;

• vitreous haemorrhage;

• advanced retinopathy with fibrous tissue or retinal detachments.

Reasons for early referral to an ophthalmologist (within 6 weeks) are:

• pre-proliferative changes;

• maculopathy;

• a fall of more than two lines on a Snellen chart.

Reasons for routine referral are:

• cataracts;

• non-proliferative retinopathy with large circinate exudates not threatening the macula/fovea;

Treatment

Glycaemic control

There is good epidemiological evidence for an association between poor glycaemic control and worsening of retinopathy, and that improving glycaemic control improves outcome:

- The Diabetes Control and Complications Trial (DCCT)[10] looked at intensive glycaemic control in type 1 patients over 6.5 years and showed a 76 per cent reduction in the risk of initially developing retinopathy in the tight glycaemic control group compared with the control group. The rate of progression of existing retinopathy was slowed by 54 per cent and the risk of developing severe non-proliferative or proliferative retinopathy was reduced by 47 per cent.

- The United Kingdom Prospective Diabetes Study (UK PDS)[4,11] looked at type 2 patients over 9 years and showed a 21 per cent reduction in progression of retinopathy and a 29 per cent reduction in the need for laser therapy in those with better glycaemic control.

The DCCT, UK PDS and several previous studies also showed an initial worsening of retinopathy in the first 2 years in the tight/improved glycaemic control groups and all patients therefore need careful monitoring over this period. This is particularly important in high-risk groups such as pregnant women. The long-term benefits, however, outweigh this initial risk.

Blood pressure control/therapy

There is good evidence for an association between both systolic and diastolic hypertension and retinopathy in type 1 patients while the link may only be with systolic hypertension in type 2 patients. The UK PDS looked at blood pressure control in type 2 patients and showed that the treatment group, with a mean blood pressure (BP) of 144/82 mmHg, when compared with a control group with a mean of 154/87 mmHg, had a 35 per cent reduction in the need for laser therapy.[12]

Adequate BP control, e.g. <140/80 in type 2 patients, is therefore advocated. Using angiotensin-converting enzyme inhibitors (ACEIs) as first-line therapy for this is also suggested. Experimental evidence suggests that these agents may have anti-angiogenic effects by altering local growth factor levels as well as any benefit from reducing blood pressure. Studies using enalapril and lisinopril have both shown a reduction in the progression of retinopathy in type 1 patients.

Lipid control/therapy

Experimental evidence suggests that oxidized low-density lipoprotein (LDL) cholesterol may be cytotoxic for endothelial cells. Epidemiological data also suggest an association between higher LDL cholesterol and worse diabetic retinopathy, especially maculopathy with exudates. A total cholesterol >7.0 mmol/l gives a fourfold greater risk of proliferative retinopathy than a total cholesterol <5.3 mmol/l. A worse outcome from laser therapy in those treated for maculopathy has also been seen if hyperlipidaemia is present. Aggressive lipid lowering is therefore advocated, especially in maculopathy.

Antiplatelet therapy

In view of the altered rheological properties of diabetic patients, these agents have been tried but the results are variable. No evidence that they make things worse has been shown and some studies suggest aspirin and ticlopidine may slow the progression of retinopathy, but the benefit is small. The other benefits of aspirin should, however, make it advisable in most patients with no contraindications.

Lifestyle advice

Although stopping smoking reduces macrovascular risk, its effect on retinopathy is less clear. Alcohol consumption and physical activity also show no consistent effect.

Potential future therapies

Current areas of research include the use of growth factor inhibitors to block IGF-1 effects and enzyme pathways utilized in hyperglycaemia, such as protein kinase beta inhibitors.

Surgical treatment

Laser treatment

Laser treatment aims to prevent further visual loss, especially in maculopathy, not to restore vision, and the distinction must be emphasized to all patients requiring treatment as this is a destructive therapy. The benefits currently outweigh the risks from laser therapy, which include blindness with accidental burns to the fovea if the eye moves during therapy, a reduction in night vision and, in a small number, interference with visual field severe enough to affect driving ability.

The ETDRS showed that laser therapy (given to one eye, with the other eye in the same patient used as a non-treated control) was better than no treatment in all visual acuity subgroups with a 24 per cent blindness rate at 3 years in the non-treated eyes compared with a 12 per cent rate in the treated group.[6]

Most patients have laser therapy performed while they are conscious, as out-patients over three to four sessions. Topical local anaesthetic drops allow a contact lens to be placed on the cornea and are often all that is needed. Alternatively a retro-orbital injection (performed through the inside of the lower eyelid), to anaesthetize the eye, can be given.

In patients with severe proliferative retinopathy, pan-retinal photocoagulation now reduces visual loss (i.e. an acuity >1/60 or worse) by over 80 per cent, while a macula grid reduces visual loss in maculopathy by over 50 per cent. Laser burns, 100–500 μm in diameter, each taking about 0.1 s to apply, are used with 1500–7000 separate burns needed for pan-retinal or 'scatter' laser photocoagulation (Figure 1.12). For oedematous/exudative maculopathy a macula grid may use only 100–200 burns of 100–200 μm diameter separated by 200–400 μm gaps, avoiding the fovea. The laser energy is absorbed by the choroid and the pigment epithelium, which lies below the neurosensory layer, also absorbing the energy/heat, and is destroyed.

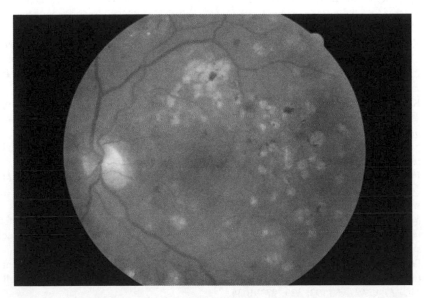

Figure 1.12 Pan-retinal photocoagulation laser therapy

Vitrectomy

If the vitreous contains scar tissue, haemorrhage or any opacity, a vitrectomy to remove it may help restore vision and aids both intra-operative and post-operative laser therapy. It can also help reduce retinal traction and allows retinal reattachment to be performed. A 70 per cent success rate for restoring vision is seen, but the risk of worsening vision, detaching the retina or worsening lens opacities should also be considered.

Cataract extraction

This is a common procedure with a slightly higher complication rate than in the non-diabetic population. Approximately 15 per cent of patients undergoing a cataract extraction can be expected to have diabetes. Worsening of maculopathy after cataract extraction is a risk, but the improved view for laser therapy outweighs this.

References

1. Evans J, Rooney C, Aswood F, Dattani N, Wormald R. Blindness and partial sight in England and Wales. *Health Trends* 1996; **38**: 5–12.
2. Klein R, Klein BEK, Moss SE. Epidemiology of proliferative diabetic retinopathy. *Diabet Care* 1992; **15**(12): 1875–1891.
3. Klein R, Klein BEK, Moss SE, Davis MD, DeMets DL. The Wisconson Epidemiological Study of Diabetic Retinopathy: II. Prevalence and risk of diabetic retinopathy when age at diagnosis is less than 30 years. *Arch Ophthal* 1984; **102**: 520–526.
4. Kohner EM, Aldington SJ, Stratton IM, Marley SE, Holman RR, Mathews DR, Turner RC. United Kingdom Prospective Diabetes Study 30. Diabetic retinopathy at diagnosis of non-insulin dependent diabetes mellitus and associated risk factors. *Arch Ophthal* 1998; **116**(3): 297–303.
5. Klein R, Klein BEK, Moss SE, Davis MD, DeMets DL. The Wisconson Epidemiological study of Diabetic Retinopathy. III. Prevalence and risk of diabetic retinopathy when age at diagnosis is 30 or more years. *Arch Ophthal* 1984; **102**: 527–532.
6. Early Treatment Diabetic Retinopathy Study Group. Early photocoagulation for diabetic retinopathy. ETDRS Report number 9. *Ophthalmology* 1991; **98**(S): 767–785.
7. Freudenstein U, Verne J. A national screening programme for diabetic retinopathy. *Br Med J* 2001; **323**: 4–5.
8. www.diabetic-retinopathy.screening.nhs.uk
9. Younis N, Broadbent DM, James M, Harding SP, Vora JP. Incidence of sight threatening retinopathy in patients with type 2 diabetes in the Liverpool diabetic eye study: a cohort study. *Lancet* 2003; **361**: 195–200.
10. DCCT Research Group. The effect of intensive treatment of diabetes on the development and treatment and progression of long-term complications in insulin dependent diabetes mellitus. *New Engl J Med* 1993; **329**: 977–1034.
11. Stratton IM, Kohner EM, Aldington SJ, Turner RC, Holman RR, Marley SE, Mathews DR. Progression of diabetic retinopathy at diagnosis of non-insulin dependent diabetes in the United Kingdom Prospective Diabetes Study. *Diabet O Logia* 2001; **44**(2): 156–163.
12. UK Prospective Diabetes Study Group. Tight blood pressure control and risk of macro-vascular and microvascular compolications in type 2 diabetes (UKPDS 38). *Br Med J* 1998; **317**: 703–712.

Useful websites

www.nice.org.uk (diabetic retinopathy: early management and screening).

www.diabetic-retinopathy.screening.nhs.uk/overview-of-screening-models.html
(preservation of sight in diabetes: a risk reduction program).

Useful addresses

The Partially Sighted Society
Queen's Road
Doncaster
DN1 2NX, UK
Tel: 01302 323132
Royal National Institute for the Blind
224 Great Portland Street
London W1, UK
Tel: 0207 3881266

Action for Blind People
14–16 Verney Road
London SE16 3DZ, UK
Tel: 0207 7328771

2
Diabetes and the Kidney

Richard J. MacIsaac and **Gerald F. Watts**

2.1 Introduction

While the introduction of insulin therapy in 1924 improved the immediate outlook for thousands of patients with diabetes mellitus, it subsequently uncovered the ogre of the long-term complications of the disease.[1] Prospective studies in diabetic clinics on both sides of the Atlantic subsequently demonstrated the high incidence rate of occlusive vascular disease, retinopathy, neuropathy and nephropathy. These are now collectively recognized to be due to a specific degenerative lesion of blood vessels referred to as diabetic angiopathy. The association between diabetes and renal disease was recognized quite early on by nineteenth-century physicians, most notably by Cotunnius and Bright. Renal disease is particularly important in diabetic patients because it provides the nexus for expression of other long-term complications of diabetes.

It has been recognized for some time that the incidence of diabetes is increasing worldwide, mainly because of an increase in type 2 diabetes. The public health impact of this phenomenon is enormous, since diabetes is now the leading cause of end-stage renal disease (ESRD) in Western countries. Diabetic nephropathy, defined as persistent clinically detectable proteinuria in association with an elevation in blood pressure and a decline in glomerular filtration rate (GFR), has been reported to occur in 25–40 per cent of people with either type 1 or type 2 diabetes. People with diabetes, especially those with renal involvement, also have an increased cardiovascular morbidity and mortality. Therefore, the early identification of people at greatest risk and the subsequent initiation of renal and cardiovascular protective treatments is of the utmost importance.

Diabetes: Chronic Complications   Edited by Kenneth M. Shaw and Michael H. Cummings
© 2005 John Wiley & Sons, Ltd.

   Microalbuminuria is an early component in a continuum of progressive increase in albumin excretion rates (AER) that usually characterizes diabetic renal disease. The term refers to a subclinical increase in urinary albumin excretion. By definition, it corresponds to an albumin excretion rate of 20–200 µg/min (30–300 mg/day) or an albumin-to-creatinine ratio (mg/mmol) of 2.5–35 in males and 3.5–35 in females (Table 2.1). The development of microalbuminuria has been equated with incipient nephropathy, but microalbuminuria is also a risk factor for macrovascular disease in people with diabetes.[2] Although recent work has suggested that a minority of subjects with diabetes and impaired renal function may not have an elevated AER, measuring albumin excretion is still the best non-invasive means of predicting and following diabetic kidney disease.[3]

Table 2.1 Classification of albuminuria for people with diabetes

	AER		ACR (mg/mmol)	
	µg/min	mg/day	Females	Males
Normoalbuminuria	<20	<30	<3.5	<2.5
Microalbuminuria	20–200	30–300	3.5–35	2.5–25
Macroalbuminuria	>200	>300	>35	>25

   This chapter will summarize the aetiology, structural and functional changes of diabetic renal disease. Clinical interventions aimed at preventing or ameliorating the progression of this devastating complication of diabetes are also outlined. Special emphasis is given to the relationship between microalbuminuria and diabetic renal disease.

2.2 Normal Renal Structure and Function

The kidney fulfils several vital functions, including the control of water and electrolyte metabolism, the regulation of arterial blood pressure and the excretion of both endogenously produced and exogenously ingested toxic chemicals. Its functional unit is the nephron, of which there are approximately 750 000 in each kidney. There is a well-recognized decline in nephron number with age. The nephron comprises a glomerulus and renal tubular system (Figure 2.1). The glomerulus consists of a capillary tuft that receives blood from the afferent arteriole (derived from the renal artery) and drains into the efferent arteriole. The wall of the glomerulus is effectively a filtration barrier, which under pressure separates blood cells and large molecules from small molecules and water. The latter form the so-called 'glomerular ultrafiltrate'. The rate at which this is formed is a measure of renal function and is referred to as the 'glomerular filtration rate'.

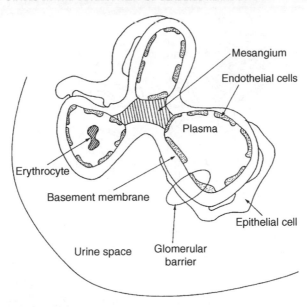

Figure 2.1 Structure of a nephron, the functional unit of the kidney. Diabetic renal disease primarily affects the glomerulus

Figure 2.2 shows in cross-section the structure of the glomerular capillary lobule of the kidney: the glomerular capillary barrier essentially consists of the inner lining of endothelial cells, the basement membrane and the outer layer of the epithelial cells; the supporting tissue or mesangium is not part of the barrier normally, but encroaches on it in diabetic glomerular disease. Pathological changes in the structure and function of the filtration barrier are reflected by changes in renal protein excretion, of which albuminuria is of most importance clinically. With an intact glomerular capillary wall, the size, shape and charge of the albumin molecule restrict its passage into the ultrafiltrate and the urine. Measurement of albumin excretion provides a useful index of the integrity of the glomerular barrier or the extent of its 'leakiness'. The renal tubular system modifies the glomerular ultrafiltrate by controlling water reabsorption in the proximal convoluted tubule, the loop of Henle, distal convoluted tubule and the collecting ducts. Given that regulation of water excretion involves other parts of the nephron, measurement of urinary AER is a better reflector of the integrity of the filtration barrier, and hence glomerular function, than measurement of urinary albumin concentration alone.

2.3 Stages in the Development of Diabetic Renal Disease

Over the last 20 years several well-defined stages in the natural history of diabetic nephropathy have been described. Diabetic renal disease is usually characterized by changes in both albuminuria and GFR in people predisposed to

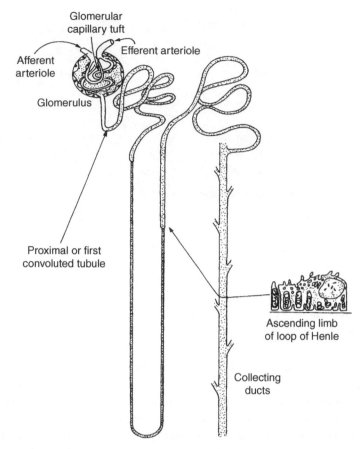

Figure 2.2 Diagrammatic high-powered cross-sectional representation of the glomerular capillary lobule of kidney. To get into the urine space, albumin has to pass from the plasma across the endothelial cells, basement membrane and epithelial cells. In diabetic renal disease the basement membrane increases in thickness and the mesangium expands to invade the glomerular barrier. Increase in albumin in the urine reflects damage to the glomerular barrier filtration rate (GFR); normal GFR ranges between 80 and 120 ml/min/1.73 m^2

the development of diabetic renal disease. The usual sequence starts with an increase in GFR ('hyperfiltration'), followed by an increase in AER leading to microalbuminuria. In parallel with these changes, there is a rise in blood pressure, which may begin before the development of microalbuminuria in type 2 diabetes, but usually occurs during the early microalbuminuric phase in type 1 diabetes. Despite this usual sequence of events, the onset of a decline in GFR may still occur in people with diabetes with minimal or no increase in albuminuria.[4]

For patients following an 'albuminuric' pathway to renal impairment, Mogensen[5] has developed a classification scheme based primarily on tests of urinary albumin excretion. The first stage is characterized by glomerular hyperfiltration and hypertrophy. Hyperfiltration, defined as a GFR above the range observed in age-matched non-diabetic subjects >135 ml/min/1.73 m^2 in young subjects), occurs in approximately 20 per cent of normoalbuminuric subjects with type 1 diabetes and 0–20 per cent of subjects with type 2 diabetes. Hyperfiltration occurs less frequently in some ethnic groups compared with others. The increase in GFR seen with hyperfiltration starts at the stage of normoalbuminuria but may continue for several years into the microalbuminuric phase. There is some evidence, especially in people with type 1 diabetes, that hyperfiltration predisposes to the development of microalbuminuria and a subsequent greater decline in GFR. The second stage consists of a 'silent phase' associated with normal urinary albumin excretion or intermittent episodes of microalbuminuria. Although the kidneys of patients with diabetes appear not to have any functional abnormalities at this stage, it is well recognized that structural changes, especially basement membrane thickening and mesangial expansion, have usually already occurred. This silent phase may last for many years and the majority of patients with diabetes will remain in this phase for their lifetime. The next phase is characterized by persistent microalbuminuria. Several studies have shown that GFR will be preserved in subjects with type 1 or type 2 diabetes during this stage as long as they remain normotensive and their AER does not begin to progressively rise. However, in type 2 diabetes, the onset of hypertension commonly precedes or accompanies this stage and subsequently promotes a rise in AER and a decline in GFR. A recent study has also suggested that an increase in systolic blood pressure during sleep may even precede the development of microalbuminuria in some people with type 1 diabetes.[6] The prevalence and significance of the finding of microalbuminuria is discussed in detail in the following section. The fourth stage, 'diabetic nephropathy', is characterized by clinically detectable proteinuria, hypertension and a subsequent decline in GFR. In untreated subjects with diabetes, GFR has been estimated to decrease by approximately 10–15 ml/min per year during this stage. In comparison, the normal age-related decline in GFR for healthy individuals is estimated to be approximately 1 ml/min per year. The final stage occurs when subjects progress to end-stage renal failure. At this stage GFR has usually decreased to below 15 ml/min, necessitating the commencement of renal replacement therapy.

The National Kidney Foundation has divided chronic renal disease into five stages based on an estimation of GFR (Table 2.2). This body has suggested

Table 2.2   Stages of chronic renal disease according to the National Kidney Foundation Disease Outcomes Quality Initiative classification

Stage	Description	GFR (ml/min/1.73 m^2)
1	Kidney damage with normal or increased GFR	$\geq$90
2	Kidney damage with a mild decrease in GFR	60–89
3	Kidney damage with a moderate decrease in GFR	30–59
4	Kidney damage with a severe decrease in GFR	15–29
5	Kidney failure	<15 (or dialysis)

that estimates of GFR are the best overall indices of the level of renal function and that GFR should be estimated from prediction equations. The preferred method is the calculation of the four-variable modified diet in renal disease (MDRD) formula:

$$\text{GFR (ml/min)}/1.73\,\text{m}^2 = 186.3 \times [1000 \times (\text{serum creatinine}/88.4)]^{-1.154}$$
$$\times (\text{age in years})^{-0.203} \times (0.742 \text{ if female})$$
$$\times (1.212 \text{ if African-American})$$

where creatinine is expressed as mmol/l. Given that AER does not always reflect GFR (see below), it is suggested that both AER and GFR are regularly estimated in subjects with type 2 diabetes.

Recent studies have suggested that there may be discordance between decrease in GFR and a rise in urinary albumin excretion in some people with diabetes, as originally described over 10 years ago.[7,8] Of 105 normoalbuminuric subjects with type 1 diabetes, 23 (22 per cent) were reported to have a GFR < 90 ml/min/ 1.73 m^2 and had advanced classical diabetic glomerular lesions. Reduced GFR and normoalbuminuria were found to be more common in females, particularly those with retinopathy or hypertension.[9] However, this relatively high prevalence of normoalbuminuria and renal insufficiency in type 1 diabetes has not been observed in other cohorts of subjects with type 1 diabetes.[10] For subjects with type 2 diabetes and a GFR < 60 ml/min/1.73 m^2, the prevalences of normo-, micro- and macroalbuminuria were reported to be 39, 35 and 26 per cent, respectively, in a recent study.[11] After accounting for the use of renin–angiotensin system (RAS) inhibitors, the prevalence of a GFR < 60 ml/min/1.73 m^2, and normoalbuminuria was still not insignificant at 23 per cent. This suggests that the relatively high prevalence of normoalbuminuric renal insufficiency was not due to regression of macro- or microalbuminuria induced by blocking the RAS. Impaired renal function and normoalbuminuria were also more common in females. Furthermore, a relatively high prevalence of renal insufficiency and normoalbuminuria in subjects with type 2 diabetes has been confirmed in a study based on results from the Third National Health and Nutrition Survey (NHANES III), which showed that 30 per cent of adults with type 2 diabetes had renal insufficiency. The authors of this latter study suggested that reduced GFR in these subjects might not be due to classic diabetic glomerulosclerosis.[12] Despite a growing awareness that GFR can still decline in normoalbuminuric patients with diabetes and a relative reduction in the number of microalbuminuric patients progressing to macroalbuminuria reported in recent studies, measurement of urinary albumin levels still appears to be the best non-invasive means of predicting and following diabetic kidney disease. However, the absence of microalbuminuria should not be interpreted to represent preservation of GFR, especially in patients with type 2 diabetes.

2.4 Prevalence and Significance of Microalbuminuria

The concept of microalbuminuria

In the early 1960s, Professor Harry Keen's Group at Guy's Hospital developed a radioimmunoassay technique for measuring very low concentrations of albumin in urine that they termed microalbuminuria, or subclinical albuminuria. This technique was employed in an epidemiological survey in Bedford, UK, in which newly diagnosed subjects with type 2 diabetes were found to have higher urinary albumin excretion than non-diabetics, and a link was reported between microalbuminuria, poor glycaemic control and high blood pressure. Interest in microalbuminuria picked up a decade or so later, and extensive work was carried out in the UK and Denmark in people with type 2 diabetes. A significant early finding was that improvement in glycaemic control with insulin could reverse microalbuminuria. Modest elevations in albumin excretion were not considered to be of major clinical importance until the early 1980s, when the finding of microalbuminuria was reported to be associated with a risk of progression to overt proteinuria of 60–80 per cent over 6–14 years.[13–16] These seminal results spawned the vast body of research now aimed at the detection and prevention of diabetic renal disease.

Prevalence, incidence, regression and progression of microalbuminuria

Microalbuminuria is a relatively common finding in the general population with a prevalence rate of around 7 per cent. The level of urinary albumin excretion has been demonstrated to be a powerful predictor of both all-cause and cardiovascular mortality in the general population, even in the absence of diabetes. Community-based surveys have suggested that the prevalence of microalbuminuria for subjects with diabetes ranges between 16 and 28 per cent.[17,18] It appears that both the absolute level and rate of progression of AER are independent predictors of all-cause mortality and renal and cardiovascular events in subjects with diabetes.

For clinic subjects with type 1 diabetes, approximately 10–20 per cent have been reported to develop microalbuminuria when followed for approximately 5–10 years. In a study from the Joslin Diabetes Centre, normoalbuminuric subjects were followed for 4 years and 11 per cent developed microalbuminuria. Subjects who smoked and had a glycated haemoglobin (A1c) of >8 per cent were at greatest risk of developing microalbuminuria.[19] At the Steno Diabetes Centre, 537 normoalbuminuric subjects were followed for a median of 9 years and 100 (18 per cent) progressed to microalbuminuria. The risk of developing microalbuminuria was associated with the duration of diabetes, with the peak risk coinciding with disease duration of 10–15 years. Baseline predictors of progression from normoalbuminuria were AER level, A1c, the presence of retinopathy and smoking.[20] A further study from this centre has demonstrated that the incidence of persistent microalbuminuria is 33.6 per cent for subjects with type 1 diabetes followed for 18 years.[21]

In contrast to type 1 diabetes, the finding of microalbuminuria is not uncommon at the time of diagnosis for subjects with type 2 diabetes. Of 782 participants in the Strong Heart Study with normal glucose tolerance and normal albuminuria at baseline, abnormal urinary albumin excretion was detected in 52 (6.6 per cent) and type 2 diabetes developed in 105 (13.4 per cent) of subjects when followed up after 3.9 years. Of those who developed diabetes, 19 (18 per cent) had an abnormal urinary albumin excretion rate, with the severity of diabetes being an important risk factor for abnormal urinary albumin excretion.[22] The importance of glycaemia in the development of microalbuminuria has also been demonstrated in the Framingham Offspring Study.[23] In this study a direct association between elevated urinary albumin excretion and fasting glucose concentrations was observed, which was apparent even when plasma glucose levels were within the normal range. In another study, 24 normoalbuminuric subjects with type 2 diabetes were followed for 7 years and seven subjects (24 per cent) were reported to develop microalbuminuria.[24] This suggests that the incidence of microalbuminuria in subjects with type 2 diabetes may be similar to that observed for type 1 diabetes.

The prognostic significance of microalbuminuria in terms of its ability to predict progression to overt nephropathy has been questioned by recent studies. In 386 subjects from the Joslin Diabetes Centre with type 1 diabetes, initially classified with microalbuminuria between 1991 and 1993 and then followed for 6 years, regression, and not progression, of microalbuminuria was reported in 58 per cent of subjects. Factors associated with regression included younger age, microalbuminuria of short duration, A1c <8.0 per cent, systolic blood pressure (BP) <115 mmHg, cholesterol <5.12 mmol/l and triglycerides <1.64 mmol/l. Interestingly, the use of angiotensin-converting enzyme inhibitors (ACEI) was not associated with regression of microalbuminuria. It was suggested by these authors that the mechanisms that underlie the beneficial effects of ACEI in preventing progression of microalbuminuria might not extend to its regression.[25] However, a Melbourne Diabetic Nephropathy Study Group investigation[26] has demonstrated a beneficial effect of ACEI in promoting regression of microalbuminuria, with regression of microalbuminuria seen in seven out of 13 (54 per cent) of normotensive subjects with type 1 diabetes treated with the ACEI perindopril, whereas no regression was observed for patients treated with the calcium-channel blocker nifedipine ($n = 10$) or placebo ($n = 10$). The reason why regression of microalbuminuria was not associated with ACEI therapy in the Joslin Diabetes Centre study remains unexplained. Furthermore, a more recent study has suggested that only 35 per cent of subjects with microalbuminuria regressed to normoalbuminuria either transiently (19 per cent) or permanently (16 per cent) when followed for 7.5 years. Also, after accounting for the use of ACEI, only 13 per cent of microalbuminuric subjects were found to spontaneously regress to normoalbuminuria.[21] The above study also suggested that 14.6 per cent of newly diagnosed subjects with type 1 diabetes followed for 18 years progressed to develop macroalbuminuria.

In a 10-year study, rates of progression of urinary albumin excretion for 5097 subjects with newly diagnosed type 2 diabetes have recently been reported by investigators from the United Kingdom Prospective Diabetes Study (UKPDS). The rate of progression from normo- to microalbuminuria was 2.0 per cent per year and from micro- to macroalbuminuria was 2.8 per cent per year. At the time of diagnosis of diabetes the prevalence of elevated urinary albumin levels, classified as microalbuminuria or worse (i.e. >50 mg/l), was 7.3 per cent and rose to approximately 25 per cent after 10 years. The prevalence of macroalbuminuria (i.e. >300 mg/l) 10 years after diagnosis was 5.3 per cent.[27] Higher rates of progression to macroalbuminuria were reported in the 1103 residents from Casale Monferrato, Italy, who had type 2 diabetes of approximately 10 years' duration and were followed for a median of 5.3 years.[28] Incidence rates per 1000 subjects for macroalbuminuria were reported as 25.8 and 53.6 for initially normo- or micro-albuminuric patients, respectively. The presence of microalbuminuria conferred a 42 per cent increased risk of progression to macroalbuminuria compared with normoalbuminuria, independent of duration or diabetes and blood pressure. Variables associated with progression to macroalbuminuria included A1c, apolipoprotein B, fibrinogen and high-density lipoprotein (HDL) cholesterol levels. Furthermore, for the 80 subjects with type 2 diabetes and microalbuminuria enrolled in the conventional treatment arm of the Steno 2 study, i.e. treated in accordance with the recommendations of the Danish Medical Association, 31 (39 per cent) progressed to macroalbuminuria with three subjects progressing to ESRD over 8 years.[29]

The above findings of improvement in the rates of regression of microalbuminuria and reduced progression to macroalbuminuria reported in some recent observational studies are not unexpected. These results do not necessarily call into question the ability of microalbuminuria to predict nephropathy but may simply reflect temporal trends in the prevention and treatment of diabetic complications in subjects with microalbuminuria.

Microalbuminuria and vascular disease

Persistent microalbuminuria is a risk factor for cardiovascular disease (CVD) in diabetic and non-diabetic subjects alike. In type 2 diabetes it is a powerful risk factor for cardiovascular mortality. Microalbuminuria reflects a generalized leakiness of vascular endothelium to macromolecules,[30] as reflected by increased transcapillary escape rate of albumin. This may reflect the so-called 'diabetes amplifier' for CVD coined by Keen. Several studies have now shown that both type 1 and type 2 diabetic patients have evidence of both endothelium-dependent, and possibly endothelium-independent, function *in vivo* of resistance and conduit arteries of the peripheral circulation.[31–33] These abnormalities represent perturbations in the biology of nitric oxide related to increased vascular oxidative stress, inflammation and accumulation of advanced glycation endproducts. Microalbuminuria in both types of diabetes is also associated with greater endothelial dysfunction,[32,33] consistent with greater expression of local and systemic vascular risk factors. Circulating risk factors aggravated by microalbuminuria include hypertension, dyslipidaemia, von Willebrand factor, fibrinogen, thrombomodulin, plasminogen activator inhibitor, soluble vascular cell adhesion molecule 1, soluble E-selectin and C-reactive protein.

As mentioned above, microalbuminuria is a strong predictor of total and CVD morbidity and mortality in patients with diabetes.[34] In an Australian study from a diabetes outpatient service, 666 patients with type 2 diabetes were followed from 1986 to 1993. For micro- compared with normoalbuminuric subjects, the hazard ratios (HR) after adjustment for age, gender and cardiovascular risk factors were 1.77 (95 per cent CI, 1.22–2.57) for all-cause and 2.34 (95 per cent CI, 1.38–3.99) for CVD mortality.[35] Not only is the presence of microalbuminuria a risk factor for CVD in subjects with diabetes, but its absolute level and rate of increase over time are predictors of CVD events. A recent study over 7 years in patients with type 2 diabetes has demonstrated that the rate of progression of AER is also an independent predictor of all-cause mortality and death from coronary heart disease (CHD).[36] For each mg/mmol per year increase in albumin-to-creatinine ratio (ACR), the HR for all-cause mortality increased by 1.67 (95 per cent CI 1.29–2.21) and for CHD increased by 4.05 (95 per cent CI 1.27–12.9) after adjustment for age, sex, duration of diabetes, smoking, A1c, lipid levels and BP. There was also a highly significant difference ($p = 0.0008$) in overall survival for patients with no or slow progression in the rate of increase in urinary albumin excretion (ACR ≤ 4 mg/mmol per year) compared with those with rapid progression (ACR > 4 mg/mmol per year). In the Micro-Hope study, the absolute level of microalbuminuria was found to be a powerful categorical risk factor for CVD events in subjects with diabetes.[37] The level of urinary albumin excretion has also been demonstrated to be a strong predictor of all-cause and cardiovascular mortality in the general population. In a study involving the residents of Groningen, a twofold increase in the urinary concentration of albumin within the microalbuminuric range was associated with a 29 per cent increase in CVD mortality, relative risk 1.29 (95 per cent CI 1.18–1.40), and a 12 per cent increase in non-CVD mortality, relative risk 1.12 (95 per cent CI 1.04–1.21). Furthermore, the risk of cardiovascular and non-cardiovascular death was even observed to increase for urinary albumin levels in the high normoalbuminuric range.[18]

2.5   Screening for Diabetic Renal Disease

Screening patients at risk for diabetic nephropathy usually involves testing for the presence of persistent microalbuminuria. Laboratory-based screening for microalbuminuria can be achieved in a number of ways:

- a 24 h urine collection for the estimation of AER, accepted as the gold standard with the added advantage of allowing for the estimation of creatinine clearance;

- a spot urine collection for the estimation of the ACR;

- a timed 4 h or overnight collection for the estimation of AER.

Alternatively, screening for microalbuminuria can be performed on spot or early morning urine samples using special reagent strips.

The reference ranges of albuminuria for AER and ACR 24 h urine collections and spot urine samples for ACR are shown in Table 2.1. At least two out of three consecutive estimations of albuminuria should fall into the microalbuminuric range before a diagnosis of persistent microalbuminuria is made. Increases in albuminuria into the microalbuminuric range may occur transiently with exercise, urinary tract infection, uncontrolled hyperglycaemia and cardiac failure (Table 2.3).[38] Care should also be taken when interpreting ACR results from

Table 2.3 Potential sources of 'false-positives' when measuring microalbuminuria

Exercise
Acute fluid intake
Haematuria
Menstrual flow
Urinary infection
Renal papillary necrosis
Semen
Urine collection error

elderly females because of false positive findings caused by low urinary creatinine levels.[39] In subjects with type 1 diabetes, it is recommended that screening for microalbuminuria commence approximately 5 years after diagnosis, as the development of diabetic complications is rare before this time. In contrast, given that approximately 20 per cent of newly diagnosed subjects with type 2 diabetes will have microalbuminuria, it is recommended that all subjects with type 2 diabetes should be screened at the time of diagnosis.

It should be remembered that the above diagnostic thresholds for microalbuminuria are arbitrary and that there is a continuous relationship between AER and clinical end-points. Even below the traditional microalbuminuria thresholds, urinary albumin levels correlate with renal and cardiovascular events, and with all-cause mortality. An algorithm for screening for microalbuminuria is shown in Figure 2.3.

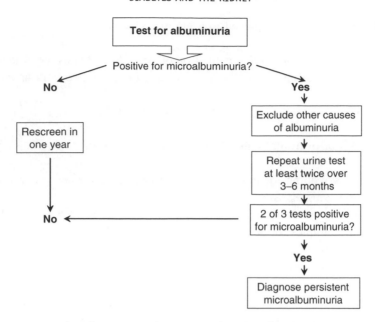

Figure 2.3   Screening strategy for microalbuminuria

2.6   Initiators and Promoters of Diabetic Renal Disease

Genetic factors clearly influence the development of diabetic renal disease.[40] Possible candidate genes are those regulating the RAS, hypertension, dyslipidaemia, hyperglycaemia and immune responses.[41] However, the role of genotyping in assessment of microalbuminuria and guiding the management of diabetic renal disease remains undefined. Family history of CHD, hypertension, renal disease and dyslipidaemia should nevertheless be routinely elicited in all diabetic patients. Candidate genes implicated in the susceptibility to the development of diabetic nephropathy are shown in Table 2.4.

Exercise-induced microalbuminuria has also been demonstrated to be predictive of later course resting microalbuminuria. Given that microalbuminuria is an indicator that the kidney is actively being damaged, undue exercise could be detrimental to early diabetic nephropathy; however, more work is required to clarify the clinical impact of exercise on the progression of microalbuminuria.[2]

The stage of microalbuminuria usually evolves over 10–15 years with defined initiators and promoters such as levels of glycaemia, blood pressure control and smoking. After the transition to the microalbuminuric or the overt nephropathy stage, the rate of progression of renal disease is influenced by a number of factors including the level of blood pressure, hyperglycaemia, the level of proteinuria or albuminuria, the presence of retinopathy, smoking and possibly anaemia. Non-modifiable risk factors include male gender and ethnicity (Table 2.5). In particular,

Table 2.4 Candidate genes implicated in the susceptibility for the development of diabetic nephropathy

Angiotensin-converting enzyme (ACE)
Angiotensinogen
Angiotensin II receptor (type 1)
Aldose reductase
Apolipoprotein E
Atrial natriuretic peptide
Heparin sulfate
Intercellular adhesion molecule-1 (ICAM)
Matrix metalloproteinase
Methylene metaloproteinase-9 (MM-9)
Na/H exchanger
Nitric oxide synthase
Plasminogen activator inhibitor-1 (PAI-1)
Peroxisome proliferator-activated receptor (PPAR)
Type 4 collagen
3-Adrenergic receptor
Vascular endothelial growth factor (VEGF)

Table 2.5 Initiators and promoters of diabetic renal disease

Initiators of DN

Hyperglycaemia
Predisposing genes

Promoters of DN

Hyperglycaemia
Hypertension
Dyslipidaemia
Insulin resistance
Smoking
Procoagulant state
Long duration of diabetes
Anaemia
Ethnicity/Westernization

higher rates of ESRD due to diabetes have been reported for Pima Indians, Mexican Americans, Asians, South Pacific Islanders, New Zealand Maoris and Australian Aborigines than for people of Caucasian origin. However, it is not clear if these inter-population differences are due to genetic changes in the predisposition to diabetic nephropathy or to environmental, social or cultural factors. The efficacy of treating modifiable initiators and promoters of diabetic renal disease is discussed in a later section.

2.7 Renal Morphology and Diabetic Nephropathy

In patients with type 1 diabetes, morphological changes occur in the renal arterioles, interstitium and tubules, but the development of a glomerulopathy is considered as the hallmark of diabetic nephropathy. This glomerulopathy is characterized by thickening of the glomerular basement membrane (GBM) and mesangial expansion. These changes have even been observed in normoalbuminuric patients, and although there is a fair degree of overlap with microalbuminuric patients, the overall severity of these changes increases with the onset of microalbuminuria. Mesangial expansion is believed to be the pathological process that leads to a decline in GFR, as it restricts the glomerular capillary lumen and reduces the filtration surface. As the ultrastructure of the glomerular epithelial cell (podocyte) has been elucidated, it has become increasingly apparent that the podocyte plays a pivotal role in the pathogenesis of albuminuria, since it is an important barrier for the trans-glomerular passage of macromolecules. This has resulted in a detailed examination of the podocyte, specifically in terms of cell number and density, in relation to AER. In subjects with type 1 diabetes, regardless of their AER status, no difference in the number of podocytes per glomerulus was found compared with control non-diabetic subjects. However, a reduction in the numerical density of podocytes per glomerulus was found in patients with type 1 diabetes and macroalbuminuria. Furthermore, glomerular basement membrane thickening has been demonstrated to be related to AER, but not GFR or the presence of hypertension, with the width of the GBM at baseline being predictive of AER after 6 years of follow-up.[42]

Compared with type 1 diabetic nephropathy, there is wider heterogeneity of renal ultrastructural morphology in type 2 diabetes. Three patterns of renal ultrastructural changes have been described for microalbuminuric patients with type 2 diabetes and preserved renal function:

(1) normal or near normal renal structure;

(2) typical diabetic glomerulopathy;

(3) three atypical patterns of renal injury – tubulo-interstitial lesions, advanced glomerular arteriolar hyalinosis and global glomerulosclerosis.

Furthermore, renal morphological changes that could be ascribed to other well-recognized forms of non-diabetic renal disease are rare.[43] At present there have been no detailed studies of renal structure in normoalbuminuric subjects with type 2 diabetes regardless of GFR. For subjects with type 2 diabetes and macroalbuminuria, three patterns of renal morphology are generally described:

(1) non-diabetic renal disease;

(2) typical diabetic glomerulopathy;

(3) atypical diabetic nephropathy with interstitial and vascular changes.

It is estimated that approximately 10–30 per cent of people with type 2 diabetes and proteinuria may have recognized forms of non-diabetic renal ultrastructural changes.

The exact relationship between albuminuria, renal morphology and progressive decreases in GFR in type 2 diabetes remains to be fully defined. One study suggested that the best predictor of the rate of decline in GFR was the severity of the glomerular structural lesion.[44] Also, subjects with typical diabetic glomerular pathology have been reported to have a greater rate of decline in GFR (5.6 vs 1.3 ml/min/1.73 m^2 per year) than subjects with non-diabetic glomerular lesions.[45] In contrast, another study found that various patterns of renal glomerular structure did not correlate with decline in GFR in microalbuminuric subjects.[46] The rate of decline of GFR for subjects with type 2 diabetes and macroalbuminuria also appears to be related to the presence of retinopathy. Subjects with retinopathy have been reported to have a faster decline in GFR than those without retinopathy (6.5 vs 1.8 ml/min/1.73 m^2 per year).[47]

2.8 Prevention and Treatment of Diabetic Renal Disease

Glycaemic control

Diabetic nephropathy does not occur in the absence of hyperglycaemia and glycaemic control is the main determinant of the onset of nephropathy. However, glycaemic control may interact with other risk factors such as hypertension, dyslipidaemia and smoking to promote the development and progression of nephropathy. The Diabetes Control and Complications Trial (DCCT) in type 1 diabetes and the UKPDS in type 2 diabetes have demonstrated the strong relationship between glycaemic control and the risk of the development of diabetic microvascular complications without a clear-cut A1c threshold. In the DCCT[48] development of microalbuminuria was reduced by 34 per cent and macroalbuminuria by 56 per cent by achieving tight glycaemic control (A1c <7.0 per cent). An interventional analysis of the UKPDS[49] demonstrated that reducing mean A1c levels from 7.9 to 7.0 per cent was associated with an absolute risk reduction of developing overt nephropathy of 11 per cent over 12 years and a risk reduction of 30 per cent for the transition from normo- to microalbuminuria in type 2 diabetes. Once the stage of overt nephropathy has been reached it is controversial whether improving glycaemic control further retards the progression of renal failure in diabetes.

Blood pressure control

In subjects with type 1 diabetes high blood pressure is usually only due to underlying diabetic renal disease and typically blood pressure only begins to increase around the time of transition from micro- to macroalbuminuria. In contrast, hypertension may be detected in approximately one-third of patients with type 2 diabetes at the time of diagnosis. In this setting the aetiology of hypertension is most likely multifactorial and possibly represents a component of the metabolic syndrome. Regardless of the sequence or underlying causes of hypertension in type 1 and type 2 diabetes, many studies have demonstrated that high blood pressure accelerates the progression of diabetic renal disease and that aggressive blood pressure lowering retards the deterioration in renal function.

Bakris et al.[50] have demonstrated that there is a relationship between achieved blood pressure and the rate of decline in GFR in clinical trials of diabetic and non-diabetic renal disease. They demonstrated that a difference in attained mean arterial pressure of 7 mmHg (MAP 107, representing 140/90 mmHg compared with MAP 100, representing 130/85 mmHg) leads to a decrease in the rate of fall in GFR from 6 to 3 ml/min per year. This indicates that the degree of blood pressure control is at least as important as the choice of drug to initiate antihypertensive therapy.

In general, the blood pressure targets for people with diabetes should be less than 130/80 mmHg. If persistent proteinuria is present, then a more stringent target of less than 120/75 is recommended. Some experts, such as Parving, have suggested that the optimal blood pressure for diabetic patients, especially those with proteinuria, is a pre-syncopal blood pressure. As discussed below, anti- hypertensive medications that interrupt the RAS appear to have renal protective effects over and above those expected from blood pressure lowering effects alone. However, achieving blood pressure goals commonly requires the combination of three or four different antihypertensive medications, especially in subjects with type 2 diabetes. People with diabetes, especially those with renal disease, are also at higher risk of CVD and therefore achieving blood pressure targets offers both renal and cardiovascular protection. It is recommended that initial antihypertensive therapy be commenced with an agent that inhibits the RAS. Diuretics are useful second agents as subjects with diabetic nephropathy commonly also have salt and water retention. If blood pressure targets are not achieved, a long-acting calcium-channel blocker should be commenced. There is a consensus that dihydropyridine calcium-channel blockers are inappropriate as first-line drugs and that they should be reserved as second-line agents and then only in combination with RAS inhibitors.[51] A β-blocker or another subgroup of a calcium-channel blocker should be prescribed if even further additional antihypertensive therapy is required. As discussed by Bakris[50] the above recommendations have to be interpreted in the context of a subject's clinical circumstances, as these may preclude certain drug combinations (e.g. the combination of β-blockers and non-dihydropyridine calcium-channel blockers), or dictate the early introduction of specific antihypertensive agents.

It also appears that the relative prognostic significance of systolic blood pressure, diastolic blood pressure and pulse pressure for predicting progression of diabetic renal disease depends on the stage of the disease. In young patients with type 1 diabetes and presumably in those with short-duration type 2 diabetes who have not reached the stage of overt diabetic nephropathy, diastolic blood pressure is a powerful predictor or renal outcomes. However, once arterial compliance is reduced, as seen with ageing and overt nephropathy, the predictive power of diastolic pressure is lost.[51]

Inhibitors of the renin–angiotensin system

In patients with diabetes, activation of the RAS produces haemodynamic and non-haemodynamic effects that contribute to the development and progression of diabetic renal disease. There is now good evidence suggesting that interrupting the RAS with an ACEI or an angiotensin receptor blocker (ARB) results in renal and cardiovascular protective effects over and above those observed by blood pressure lowering alone. In a landmark trial, Lewis et al.[52] demonstrated that captopril reduced the risk of achieving the combined endpoint of death, dialysis and transplantation compared with blood pressure control alone achieved with non-RAS blocking agents in subjects with type 1 diabetes and macroalbuminuria. In another important study, captopril significantly reduced the progression from micro- to macroalbuminuria and prevented an increase in AER in patients with type 1 diabetes.[53] A subsequent systematic review of the effects of ACEI in patients traditionally classified as normotensive, who also had microalbuminuria, has been performed.[54] It concluded that ACEI use significantly reduced the progression to macroalbuminuria and increased the chances of remission to normoalbuminuria. The beneficial effects of ACEI were observed to be weakest at the lowest levels of microalbuminuria but did not differ according to other baseline risk factors.

For subjects with type 2 diabetes and one other cardiovascular risk factor, the ACEI ramipril reduced cardiovascular events by 25 per cent and the progression to overt nephropathy by 24 per cent in 3577 patients enrolled in the Micro-HOPE study.[37] Given that these results were achieved with only a 2.4/1.0 mmHg decrease in clinic blood pressure recordings, the cardiovascular effects of ramipril were mainly considered to be independent of blood pressure lowering. In the Irbesartan Microalbuminuria Type 2 Diabetes Mellitus trial (IRMA2), irbesartan had renoprotective effects in hypertensive patients with type 2 diabetes and microalbuminuria that were reported to be greater than that attributable to blood pressure lowering alone.[55] This end-organ protective effect also appeared to be dose-dependent. Furthermore, an ambulatory blood pressure study in a subgroup from this cohort has confirmed that the beneficial effect of irbesartan on albumin excretion could not be explained by a reduction in blood pressure alone. Valsartan has also been shown to reduce albuminuria, independent of its blood pressure lowering actions, in hypertensive and normotensive subjects with type 2 diabetes and microalbuminuria.[56] More recently, losartan was shown to produce a significant reduction in urinary albumin excretion in subjects with type 2 diabetes and microalbuminuria,[57] who would have been classified as normotensive under the current criteria proposed by either the World Health Organization–International Society of Hypertension (WHO-ISH) or Joint National Committee on Prevention, Detection, Evaluation and Treatment of High Blood Pressure (JNC-7) guidelines (mean baseline blood pressure 135.9/78.8 mmHg in the losartan treated group). This suggests that normotensive subjects with type 2 diabetes and microalbuminuria should also possibly be treated with agents that interrupt the RAS. Despite these findings, preventing even small increases in blood pressure in non-hypertensive patients with type 2 diabetes and microalbuminuria, regardless of whether this involves RAS blockade, appears to stabilize AER and attenuate a decline in GFR in proportion to decrease in blood pressure.[71]

For subjects with type 2 diabetes, hypertension and macroalbuminuria, the Irbesartan Diabetic Nephropathy Trial (IDNT)[58] demonstrated that, compared with amlodipine treatment, irbesartan produced a 23 per cent relative risk reduction in the primary composite end-point of a doubling of creatinine concentration, development of end-stage renal disease and death from any cause ($p < 0.006$). This difference was observed for similar on-treatment MAP readings. In a similar population, the Reductions in Endpoints in Non-Insulin Dependent Diabetes Mellitus with the Angiotensin II Antagonist Losartan (RENAAL) study[59] showed that, compared with a placebo-treated group not receiving RAS inhibitors, losartan reduced the risk of a doubling of serum creatinine by 25 per cent ($p = 0.006$) and the progression to end-stage renal disease (ESRD) by 25 per cent ($p = 0.002$). In the IDNT and RENAAL trials, treatment with an ARB did not reduce mortality, but losartan significantly reduced the risk of hospitalization for heart failure compared with placebo. However, there is also evidence that ARB treatment can provide cardiovascular protection in subjects with diabetes. In a subgroup of subjects in the Losartan Intervention for Endpoint Reduction in Hypertension study (Diab-LIFE) who had diabetes, losartan vs atenolol treatment resulted in a 24 per cent risk reduction ($p = 0.031$) in the primary endpoint of cardiovascular death, stroke or myocardial infarction, despite similar reductions in blood pressure being achieved.[60] In contrast, a meta-analysis of the IDNT, RENAAL and Diab-LIFE studies failed to show that ARB treatment led to a significant reduction in total mortality and cardiovascular mortality.[61]

There has been some debate as to whether an ARB or an ACEI should be used as first line therapy for RAS blockade in patients with type 2 diabetes. Two recent trials have strengthened the case for ACEI use. In the BENEDICT (Bergamo Nephrologic Diabetes Complication) trial, the use of the ACEI trandolapril attenuated the progression from normoalbuminuria to microalbuminuria in subects with type 2 diabetes and hypertension. The unique protective effects of RAS blockade in hypertensive patients was emphasized as the calcium channel blocker verapamil did not prevent the onset of microalbuminuria.[72] An ACEI enalapril has also been demonstrated to provide equivalent long-term renoprotection compared to the ARB telmisartan, as measured by a decline in GFR, in hypertensive patients with type 2 diabetes and early nephropathy.[73]

Both ARBs and ACEI use may prove to have equivalent beneficial effects as first-line therapy in subjects with type 2 daibetes but the question as to which agent to use may, to some extent, be academic as many patients will possibly end up being treated with the early introduction of both agents.

Dual blockade of the RAS with an ACEI and ARB in subjects with type 2 diabetes and microalbuminuria has been demonstrated to be more effective in reducing blood pressure and decreasing albuminuria than either agent as monotherapy.[62] In macroalbuminuric patients with type 1 and type 2 diabetes, the addition of an ARB to ACEI therapy has been reported to provide superior renoprotection in terms of reducing albuminuria compared with maximal recommended doses of an ACEI in type 1 and type 2 diabetes. Whether the effects of dual therapy with an ACEI and an ARB will ultimately translate to a reduced incidence of ESRD in patients with diabetes is unknown. However, the recent COOPERATE study from Japan demonstrated that dual therapy in non-diabetic proteinuric patients was superior to monotherapy in retarding progression to ESRD, despite similar blood pressures in the different treatment groups.[63] Combining an ACEI with a diuretic or a calcium-channel blocker may also produce greater reductions in AER than monotherapy with an ACEI. In addditon, salt restriction appears to potentiate the effects of interruption of the RAS in reducing albuminuria in hypertensive subjects with type 2 diabetes.

Lipid regulation

Several observational studies, both cross-sectional and follow-up, have shown associations between dyslipoproteinaemia, specifically elevation in apoB-100-containing lipoproteins and low HDL, and albuminuria in subjects with diabetes.[64,65] Two interventional studies have shown that treatment with HMG-CoA reductase inhibitors significantly decreases AER in microalbuminuric subjects with type 2 diabetes. In contrast, simvastatin was not shown to alter AER or GFR in a 36-week placebo-controlled study of 18 subjects with type 2 diabetes, microalbuminuria and cholesterol levels equal or greater than 5.5 mmol/l. Similar effects have not been observed for interventional studies involving subjects with type 1 diabetes. It is important to emphasize that intensive treatment of dyslipidaemia in people with diabetes should be considered not only to ameliorate renal injury but also to avoid cardiovascular complications.[66] As indicated earlier, endothelial dysfunction is a feature of microalbuminuria in diabetes. It has been recently shown in a controlled trial that atorvastatin (40 mg/day) improved both endothelium-dependent and endothelium-independent vasodilator function of the brachial artery in type 1 diabetic patients with microalbuminuria.[67] These improvements were, however, unrelated to changes in plasma lipid levels and could reflect the so-called 'pleiotropic effects' of statins such as reduction in oxidative stress and vascular inflammation. There may be a case for treating all diabetic patients with microalbuminuria with statins, but this needs to be confirmed with clinical outcome data.

Smoking cessation

Several observational studies have documented an association between smoking and diabetic nephropathy. However, no studies have assessed the renal effects of smoking cessation. In particular, smoking appears to promote the initiation of microalbuminuria and the subsequent transition to macroalbuminura. There is some evidence to suggest that cessation of smoking retards the progression of diabetic nephropathy in type 1 diabetes. A similar effect is likely for subjects with type 2 diabetes. Smoking is already an established risk factor for CVD and may possibly also play a role in the onset and progression of diabetic nephropathy. Even though there is a lack of definitive interventional studies for smoking, the above evidence provides a strong rationale for the inclusion of smoking cessation in the management of subjects with type 2 diabetes and microalbuminuria.

Protein restriction

Although the relationship between a high protein intake and the risk of onset and progression of diabetic renal disease is not conclusive, a meta-analysis has demonstrated that protein restriction in patients with type 1 diabetes and overt nephropathy slows the rate of decline in GFR. A single study of subjects with type 1 diabetes and microalbuminuria also concluded that the rate of progression to overt nephropathy was slowed by protein restriction. In a more recent study of subjects with type 1 diabetes and progressive diabetic nephropathy, the relative risk of ESRD or death was 0.23 (95 per cent CI 0.07–0.72, $p = 0.01$) for patients assigned to moderate dietary protein restriction (0.89 g/kg per day) compared with those assigned to a usual protein diet (1.02 g/kg per day).[68] Interestingly, despite this difference in event rates, the decline in GFR in the two groups was similar. The American Diabetes Association guidelines for the management of diabetic nephropathy now recommend prescribing a protein intake of 0.8 g/kg per day in subjects with overt nephropathy.[69]

Correction of anaemia

Anaemia is common in patients with diabetes and is emerging as a potential risk factor for the progression of diabetic renal disease.[70] At present it is not known whether the potential benefits of correcting anaemia with erythropoietin outweigh the risks of hypertension and the possible worsening of anaemia due to red cell aplasia. Clinical trails are currently in progress to answer these questions.

2.9 Summary and Clinical Recommendations

In summary, screening people with diabetes for early markers of diabetic renal disease and initiation of measures to retard the progression of diabetic nephropathy are now considered part of routine clinical practice. In addition it is necessary to measure, assess and manage cardiovascular risk factors aggressively. We recommend that annual screening for microalbuminuria be performed in people who have had type 1 diabetes for at least 5 years and in those with type 2 diabetes starting at the time of diagnosis. In particular, the finding of microalbuminuria should provoke an intensified modification of the common risk factors for renal and CVD, i.e. hyperglycaemia, hypertension, dyslipidaemia and smoking. Antihypertensive therapy in people with diabetes should be initiated with an ACEI or an ARB. A suggested treatment strategy for people with diabetes and microalbuminuria is shown in Figure 2.4. It has been shown that multi-interventional, target-driven strategies, aiming for an A1c <6.5 per cent, systolic blood pressure <130 mmHg, diastolic blood pressure <80 mmHg, fasting cholesterol <4.5 mmol/l and fasting triglycerides <1.7 mmol/l, that includes the universal use of ACEI and aspirin and the aggressive use of statins, decreases cardiovascular and microvascular events by approximately 50 per cent in people with type 2 diabetes and microalbuminuria.[29] Subjects with diabetes and microalbuminuria should be managed by diabetologists or physicians experienced in modifying the common risk factors for renal and CVD. In general, subjects with a GFR <30 ml/min/ 1.73 m^2 should be referred to a nephrologist in preparation for the commencement of renal replacement therapy.

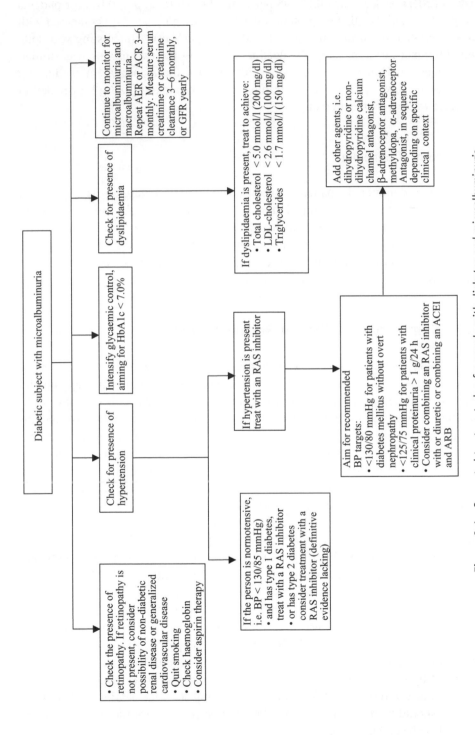

Figure 2.4 Suggested treatment plan for people with diabetes and microalbuminuria

References

1. Nathan DM. Long-term complications of diabetes mellitus. *New Engl J Med* 1993; **328**: 1676–1685.

2. Watts GF, Jasik M, Cooper ME. The implications of the detection of proteinuria and microalbuminuria in insulin and non-insulin dependent diabetes. *Aust NZ J Med* 1995; **25**: 157–161.

3. Caramori ML, Fioretto P, Mauer M. The need for early predictors of diabetic nephropathy risk: is albumin excretion rate sufficient? *Diabetes* 2000; **49**: 1399–1408.

4. MacIsaac RJ, Jerums G, Cooper ME. New insights into the significance of microalbuminuria. *Curr Opin Nephrol Hypertens* 2004; **13**: 83–91.

5. Mogensen CE. Microalbuminuria, blood pressure and diabetic renal disease: origin and development of ideas. *Diabetologia* 1999; **42**: 263–285.

6. Lurbe E, Redon J, Kesani A, Pascual JM, Tacons J, Alvarez V, Batlle D. Increase in nocturnal blood pressure and progression to microalbuminuria in type 1 diabetes. *New Engl J Med* 2002; **347**: 797–805.

7. Lane PH, Steffes MW, Mauer SM. Glomerular structure in IDDM women with low glomerular filtration rate and normal urinary albumin excretion *Diabetes* 1992; **41**: 581–586.

8. Tsalamandris C, Allen TJ, Gilbert RE, Sinha A, Panagiotopoulos S, Cooper ME, Jerums G. Progressive decline in renal function in diabetic patients with and without albuminuria. *Diabetes* 1994; **43**: 649–655.

9. Caramori ML, Fioretto P, Mauer M. Low glomerular filtration rate in normoalbuminuric type 1 diabetic patients: an indicator of more advanced glomerular lesions. *Diabetes* 2003; **52**: 1036–1040.

10. Hansen KW, Mau Pedersen M, Christensen CK, Schmitz A, Christiansen JJ, Mogensen CE. Normoalbuminuria ensures no reduction of renal function in type 1 (insulin-dependent) diabetic patients. *J Intern Med* 1992; **232**: 161–167.

11. MacIsaac RJ, Tsalamandris C, Panagiotopoulos S, Smith TJ, McNeil KJ, Jerums G. Nonalbuminuric renal insufficiency in type 2 diabetes. *Diabet Care* 2004; **27**: 195–200.

12. Kramer HJ, Nguyen QD, Curhan G, Hsu CY. Renal insufficiency in the absence of albuminuria and retinopathy among adults with type 2 diabetes mellitus. *JAMA* 2003; **289**: 3273–3277.

13. Parving HH, Oxenboll B, Svendsen PA, Christiansen JS, Andersen AR. Early detection of patients at risk of developing diabetic nephropathy. A longitudinal study of urinary albumin excretion. *Acta Endocrinol (Copenh)* 1982; **100**: 550–555.

14. Viberti GC, Jarrett RJ, Mahmud U, Hill RD, Argyropoulos A, Keen H. Microalbuminuria as a predictor of clinical nephropathy in insulin-dependent diabetes mellitus. *Lancet* 1982; **1**: 1430–1432.

15. Mathiesen ER, Oxenboll B, Johansen K, Vendsen PA, Deckert T. Incipient nephropathy in type 1 (insulin-dependent) diabetes. *Diabetologia* 1984; **26**: 406–410.

16. Mogensen CE, Christensen CK. Predicting diabetic nephropathy in insulin-dependent patients. *New Engl J Med* 1984; **311**: 89–93.

17. Jones CA, Francis ME, Eberhardt MS, Chavers B, Coresh J, Engelgam M, Kusek JW, Byrd-Holt D, Narayan KM, Herman WH, Jones CP, Salive M, Agodoa LY. Microalbuminuria in the US population: third National Health and Nutrition Examination Survey. *Am J Kidney Dis* 2002; **39**: 445–459.

18. de Jong PE, Hillege HL, Pinto-Sietsma SJ, de Zeeuw D. Screening for microalbuminuria in the general population: a tool to detect subjects at risk for progressive renal failure in an early phase? *Nephrol Dial Transplant* 2003; **18**: 10–13.

19. Scott LJ, Warram JH, Hanna LS, Lattel LM, Ryan L, Krolewski AS. A nonlinear effect of hyperglycemia and current cigarette smoking are major determinants of the onset of microalbuminuria in type 1 diabetes. *Diabetes* 2001; **50**: 2842–2849.
20. Rossing P, Hougaard P, Parving HH. Risk factors for development of incipient and overt diabetic nephropathy in type 1 diabetic patients: a 10-year prospective observational study. *Diabet Care* 2002; **25**: 859–864.
21. Hovind P, Tarnow L, Rossing P, Jensen BR, Graae M, Torp I, Binder C, Parving HH. Predictors for the development of microalbuminuria and macroalbuminuria in patients with type 1 diabetes: inception cohort study. *Br Med J* 2004; **328**: 1105.
22. Sosenko JM, Hu D, Welty T, Howard Br, Lee E, Robbins DC. Albuminuria in recent-onset type 2 diabetes: the Strong Heart Study. *Diabet Care* 2002; **25**: 1078–1084.
23. Meigs JB, D'Agostino RB Sr, Nathan DM, Ritai N, Wilson PW. Longitudinal association of glycemia and microalbuminuria: the Framingham Offspring Study. *Diabet Care* 2002; **25**: 977–983.
24. Tabaei BP, Al-Kassab AS, Ilag LL, Zawacki CM, Herman WH. Does microalbuminuria predict diabetic nephropathy? *Diabet Care* 2001; **24**: 1560–1566.
25. Perkins BA, Ficociello LH, Silva KH, Finkelstein DM, Warram JH, Krolewski AS. Regression of microalbuminuria in type 1 diabetes. *New Engl J Med* 2003; **348**: 2285–2293.
26. Jerums G, Allen TJ, Campbell DJ, Cooper ME, Gilbert RE, Hammond JJ, Raffaele J, Tsalamandris C. Long-term comparison between perindopril and nifedipine in normotensive patients with type 1 diabetes and microalbuminuria. *Am J Kidney Dis* 2001; **37**: 890–899.
27. Adler AI, Stevens RJ, Manley SE, Bilous RW, Cull CA, Holman RR. Development and progression of nephropathy in type 2 diabetes: the United Kingdom Prospective Diabetes Study (UKPDS 64). *Kidney Int* 2003; **63**: 225–232.
28. Bruno G, Merletti F, Biggeri A, Bargero G, Ferrero S, Pagano G, Cavallo Perin P. Progression to overt nephropathy in type 2 diabetes: the Casale Monferrato Study. *Diabet Care* 2003; **26**: 2150–2155.
29. Gaede P, Vedel P, Larsen N, Jensen GV, Parving HH, Pedersen O. Multifactorial intervention and cardiovascular disease in patients with type 2 diabetes. *New Engl J Med* 2003; **348**: 383–393.
30. Deckert T, Feldt-Rasmussen B, Borch-Johnsen K, Jensen T, Kofoed-Enevoldsen A. Albuminuria reflects widespread vascular damage. The Steno hypothesis. *Diabetologia* 1989; **32**: 219–226.
31. Watts GF, Playford DA (1998). Dyslipoproteinaemia and hyperoxidative stress in the pathogenesis of endothelial dysfunction in non-insulin dependent diabetes mellitus: an hypothesis. *Atherosclerosis* 1998; **141**: 17–30.
32. Dogra G, Rich L, Stanton K, Watts GF. Endothelium-dependent and independent vasodilation studies at normoglycaemia in type I diabetes mellitus with and without microalbuminuria. *Diabetologia* 2001; **44**: 593–601.
33. Stehouwer CD, Gall MA, Twisk JW, Knudsen E. Emeris JJ, Parving HH. Increased urinary albumin excretion, endothelial dysfunction, and chronic low-grade inflammation in type 2 diabetes: progressive, interrelated, and independently associated with risk of death. *Diabetes* 2002; **51**: 1157–1165.
34. Dinneen SF, Gerstein HC. The association of microalbuminuria and mortality in non-insulin-dependent diabetes mellitus. A systematic overview of the literature. *Arch Intern Med* 1997; **157**: 1413–1418.
35. Beilin J, Stanton KG, McCann VJ, Knuiman MW, Divitini ML. Microalbuminuria in type 2 diabetes: an independent predictor of cardiovascular mortality. *Aust NZ J Med* 1996; **26**: 519–525.

36. Spoelstra-de Man AM, Brouwer CB, Stehouwer CD, Smulders YM. Rapid progression of albumin excretion is an independent predictor of cardiovascular mortality in patients with type 2 diabetes and microalbuminuria. *Diabet Care* 2001; **24**: 2097–2101.

37. HOPE. Effects of ramipril on cardiovascular and microvascular outcomes in people with diabetes mellitus: results of the HOPE study and MICRO-HOPE substudy. Heart Outcomes Prevention Evaluation Study Investigators. *Lancet* 2000; **355**: 253–259.

38. Watts GF, Kubal C, Chinn S. Long-term variation of urinary albumin excretion in insulin-dependent diabete mellitus: some practical recommendations for monitoring microalbuminuria. *Diabete Res Clin Pract* 1990; **9**: 169–177.

39. Houlihan CA, Tsalamandris C, Akdeniz A, Jerums G. Albumin to creatinine ratio: a screening test with limitations. *Am J Kidney Dis* 2002; **39**: 1183–1189.

40. Seaquist ER, Goetz FC, Rich S, Barbosa J. Familial clustering of diabetic kidney disease. Evidence for genetic susceptibility to diabetic nephropathy. *New Engl J Med* 1989; **320**: 1161–1165.

41. Thomas MC. Inherited susceptibility to diabetic nephropathy. In *Management of Diabetic Nephropathy*, Boner G and Cooper M (eds). Martin Dunitz: London, 2004; 61–73.

42. Dalla Vestra M, Saller A, Bortoloso E, Mauer M, Fioretto P. Structural involvement in type 1 and type 2 diabetic nephropathy. *Diabet Metab* 2000; **26** (suppl. 4): 8–14.

43. Fioretto P, Mauer M, Brocco E, Velussi M, Frigato F, Muollo B, Sambataro M, Abaterusso C, Baggio B, Crepaldi G, Nosadini R. Patterns of renal injury in NIDDM patients with microalbuminuria. *Diabetologia* 1996; **39**: 1569–1576.

44. Nosadini R, Velussi M, Brocco E, Bruseghin M, Abaterusso C, Saller A, Dalla Vestra M, Carraro A, Bortoloso E, Sambataro M, Barzon I, Frigato F, Muollo B, Chiesura-Corona M, Pacini G, Baggio B, Piarulli F, Sfriso A, Fioretto P. Course of renal function in type 2 diabetic patients with abnormalities of albumin excretion rate. *Diabetes* 2000; **49**: 476–484.

45. Christensen PK, Gall MA, Parving HH. Course of glomerular filtration rate in albuminuric type 2 diabetic patients with or without diabetic glomerulopathy. *Diabet Care* 2000; **23** (suppl. 2): B14–20.

46. Ruggenenti P, Gambara V, Perna A, Bertani T, Remuzzi G. The nephropathy of non-insulin-dependent diabetes: predictors of outcome relative to diverse patterns of renal injury. *J Am Soc Nephrol* 1998; **9**: 2336–2343.

47. Trevisan R, Vedovato M, Mazzon C, Coracina A, Iori E, Tiergo A, Del Prato S. Concomitance of diabetic retinopathy and proteinuria accelerates the rate of decline of kidney function in type 2 diabetic patients. *Diabet Care* 2002; **25**: 2026–2031.

48. DCCT. The effect of intensive treatment of diabetes on the development and progression of long-term complications in insulin-dependent diabetes mellitus. The Diabetes Control and Complications Trial Research Group. *New Engl J Med* 1993; **329**: 977–986.

49. UKPDS. Intensive blood-glucose control with sulphonylureas or insulin compared with conventional treatment and risk of complications in patients with type 2 diabetes (UKPDS 33). UK Prospective Diabetes Study (UKPDS) Group. *Lancet* 1998; **352**: 837–853.

50. Bakris GL, Williams M, Dworkin L, Elliott WJ, Epstein M, Toto R, Tuttle K, Douglas J, Hsueh W, Sowers J. Preserving renal function in adults with hypertension and diabetes: a consensus approach. National Kidney Foundation Hypertension and Diabetes Executive Committees Working Group. *Am J Kidney Dis* 2000; **36**: 646–661.

51. Bakris GL, Weir MR, Shanifar S, Zhang Z, Douglas J, van Dijk DJ, Brenner BM. Effects of blood pressure level on progression of diabetic nephropathy: results from the RENAAL study. *Arch Intern Med* 2003; **163**: 1555–1565.

52. Lewis EJ, Hunsicker LG, Bain RP, Rohde RD. The effect of angiotensin-converting-enzyme inhibition on diabetic nephropathy. The Collaborative Study Group. *New Engl J Med* 1993; **329**: 1456–1462.

53. Viberti G, Mogensen CE, Groop LC, Pauls JF. Effect of captopril on progression to clinical proteinuria in patients with insulin-dependent diabetes mellitus and microalbuminuria. European Microalbuminuria Captopril Study Gro up. *JAMA* 1994; **271**: 275–279.

54. ACE Inhibitors in Diabetic Nephropathy Trialist Group. Should all patients with type 1 diabetes mellitus and microalbuminuria receive angiotensin-converting enzyme inhibitors? A meta-analysis of individual patient data. *Ann Intern Med* 2001; **134**: 370–379.

55. Parving HH, Lehnert H, Brochner-Mortensen J, Gomis R, Andersen S, Arner P. The effect of irbesartan on the development of diabetic nephropathy in patients with type 2 diabetes. *New Engl J Med* 2001; **345**: 870–878.

56. Viberti G, Wheeldon NM. Microalbuminuria reduction with valsartan in patients with type 2 diabetes mellitus: a blood pressure-independent effect. *Circulation* 2002; **106**: 672–678.

57. Zandbergen AA, Baggen MG, Lamberts SW, Bootsma KH, de Zeeuw D, Ouwendijk RJ. Effect of losartan on microalbuminuria in normotensive patients with type 2 diabetes mellitus. A randomized clinical trial. *Ann Intern Med* 2003; **139**: 90–96.

58. Lewis EJ, Hunsicker LG, Clarke WR, Berl T, Pohl MA, Lewis JB, Ritz E, Atkins RC, Rohde R, Raz I. Renoprotective effect of the angiotensin-receptor antagonist irbesartan in patients with nephropathy due to type 2 diabetes. *New Engl J Med* 2001; **345**: 851–860.

59. Brenner BM, Cooper ME, de Zeeuw D, Keane WF, Mitch WE, Parving HH, Remuzzi G, Snappin SM, Zhang Z, Shahinfar S. Effects of losartan on renal and cardiovascular outcomes in patients with type 2 diabetes and nephropathy. *New Engl J Med* 2001; **345**: 861–869.

60. Lindholm LH, Ibsen H, Dahlof B, Devrrux RB, Beevers G, de Faire U, Fyhrquist F, Julius S, Kjeldsen SE, Kristiansson K, Lederballe-Pedersen O, Nieminen MS, Omvik P, Oparil S, Wedel H, Arup. Cardiovascular morbidity and mortality in patients with diabetes in the Losartan Intervention For Endpoint reduction in hypertension study (LIFE): a randomised trial against atenolol. *Lancet* 2002; **359**: 1004–1010.

61. Siebenhofer A, Plank J, Horvath K, Berghold A, Sutton AJ, Sommer R, Pieber TR. Angiotensin receptor blockers as anti-hypertensive treatment for patients with diabetes mellitus: meta-analysis of controlled double-blind randomized trials. *Diabet Med* 2004; **21**: 18–25.

62. Mogensen CE, Neldam S, Tikkanen I, Oren S, Viskoper R, Watts RW, Cooper ME. Randomised controlled trial of dual blockade of renin-angiotensin system in patients with hypertension, microalbuminuria, and non-insulin dependent diabetes: the candesartan and lisinopril microalbuminuria (CALM) study. *Br Med J* 2000; **321**: 1440–1444.

63. Nakao N, Yoshimura A, Morita H, Takada M, Kayaro T, Ideura T. Combination treatment of angiotensin-II receptor blocker and angiotensin-converting-enzyme inhibitor in non-diabetic renal disease (COOPERATE): a randomised controlled trial. *Lancet* 2003; **361**: 117–124.

64. Watts GF, Naumova R, Slavin BM, Morris RW, Houlston R, Kubal C, Shaw KM. Serum lipids and lipoproteins in insulin-dependent diabetic patients with persistent microalbuminuria. *Diabet Med* 1989; **6**: 25–30.

65. Watts GF, Powrie JK, O'Brien SF, Shaw KM. Apolipoprotein B independently predicts progression of very-low-level albuminuria in insulin-dependent diabetes mellitus. *Metabolism* 1996; **45**: 1101–1107.

66. Jandeleit-Dahm K, Bonnet F. Treatment of diabetic nephropathy: control of serum lipids. In *Management of Diabetic Nephropathy*, Boner G and Cooper M (eds). Martin Dunitz: London, 2003; 135–141.

67. Dogra GK, Watts GF, Herrmann S. Statin therapy improves brachial artery endothelial function in nephrotic syndrome. *Kidney Int* 2002; **62**: 550–557.

68. Hansen HP, Tauber-Lassen E, Jensen BR, Parving HH. Effect of dietary protein restriction on prognosis in patients with diabetic nephropathy. *Kidney Int* 2002; **62**: 220–228.

69. Molitch ME, DeFronzo RA, Franz MJ, Keane WF, Mogensen CE, Parving HH, Steffes MW. Nephropathy in diabetes. *Diabet Care* 2004; **27** (suppl. 1): S79–83.
70. Thomas MC, MacIsaac RJ, Tsalamandris C, Power D, Jerums G. Unrecognized anemia in patients with diabetes: a cross-sectional survey. *Diabet Care* 2003; **26**: 1164–1169.
71. Jerums G, Allen TJ, Campbell DJ, Cooper ME, Gilbert RE, Hammond JJ, O'Brien RC, Raffaele J, Tsalamandris C. Long-term renoprotection by perindopril or nifedipine in non-hypertensive patients with type 2 diabetes and microalbuminuria. *Diabet Med* 2004; **21**: 1192–1199.
72. Ruggenenti P, Fassi A, Ilieva AP, Bruno S, Iliev IP, Brusegan V, Rubis N, Gherardi G, Arnoldi F, Ganeva M, Ene-Iordache B, Gaspari F, Perna A, Bossi A, Trevisan R, Dodesini AR, Remuzzi G for the Bergamo Nephrologic Diabetes Complication Trial (BENEDICT) Investigators. Preventing microalbuminuria in type 2 diabetes. *New Engl J Med* 2004; **351**: 1941–1951.
73. Barnett AH, Bain SC, Bouter P, Karlberg B, Madsbad S, Jervell J, Mustonen J for the Diabetics Exposed to Telmisartan and Enalapril Study Group. Angiotensin-receptor blockade versus converting-enzyme inhibition in type 2 diabetes and nephropathy. *New Engl J Med* 2004; **35**: 1952–1961.

3

Diabetes and Foot Disease

Darryl Meeking, **Emma Holland** and **Deborah Land**

3.1   Introduction

No discussion of diabetic foot disease can be complete without acknowledging the
significant impact that this complication has in terms of its cost to the health
economy and its effects on the mortality and morbidity of those with diabetes.[1,2]
Foot ulceration in diabetes is common. In the UK diabetic population its
prevalence is likely to be between 5 and 7.4 per cent.[1,3,4] Despite this, diabetic
foot disease is an area that has been poorly studied. As a consequence, there is a
lack of agreement, let alone consensus, on how best to prevent, investigate and
manage the major diabetic foot conditions.

This chapter aims to provide an understanding of the spectrum of foot
complications associated with diabetes and to give practical guidelines for the
management of each condition at different stages of its development.

We have, not unexpectedly, chosen to focus upon diabetic foot ulceration, its
development, management and associated complications. Neuropathic pain and its
management receives significant coverage since we believe this to be a poorly
understood problem that causes significant morbidity and for which management
strategies are poorly developed and often inadequately applied.

We have also incorporated a section on Charcot deformity. This is a condition
that frequently remains unrecognized or misdiagnosed until significant damage has
occurred.

We finish by focussing upon the organization and provision of foot care and
have attempted to provide an insight into the key individuals who should take a
lead in the area. We make no apologies for making mention of the multidisciplinary foot care *team* rather than the multidisciplinary foot *clinic*. It is

Diabetes: Chronic Complications   Edited by Kenneth M. Shaw and Michael H. Cummings
© 2005 John Wiley & Sons, Ltd.

clear to us that such a clinic is not practical in all clinical settings but there are other systems that can be used to help manage patients with diabetic foot disease.

In composing this chapter there have been contributions from a range of specialists dealing with patients who suffer with diabetic foot disease (predominantly a specialist physician, specialist nurse and specialist podiatrist).

3.2 Diabetic Foot Ulceration

There are a number of factors associated with the development of diabetic foot ulceration. It is caused by one or more of three major risk factors: abnormal foot shape, nerve damage (neuropathy) and impairment of blood supply.

Abnormal foot shape

Foot deformities lead to differing pressure loads within the feet. Localized high-pressure areas are caused by abnormal bony prominences. In the neuropathic foot, elevated local pressure increases the likelihood of hyperkeratosis and subsequent callus formation. Callus formation causes a further elevation in plantar pressure[5] and this can eventually lead to ulceration. Where the blood supply to the foot is impaired, excessive pressures can lead directly to foot tissue damage and subsequent ulceration. Deformities in the diabetic foot may be due in part to limitation of joint mobility. There is abnormal glycosylation of connective tissue that in turn leads to limitation of joint movement and functional foot problems.

Normalizing foot function is important in preserving normal plantar pressures during walking. There are a number of common joint deformities.

Hallux rigidus is a condition where excessive plantar pressures are created by increased structural or functional stiffness in the first metatarso-phalangeal joint. In the deformity known as *pes cavus* there are increased pressure loads under the metatarsal heads. This condition is due to excessive concavity of the medial longitudinal arch that stretches between the calcaneus and first metatarsal head.

Ankle equinus leads to increased pressures beneath the forefoot and is due to reduced mobility of the ankle joint.

Claw or hammer toes lead to increased pressure loads beneath the metatarsal heads and at the tips of the toes on the plantar surface. Callus formation and abrasions can also occur over the dorsal surfaces of interphalangeal joints. This condition occurs as a result of hyperextension of the metatarso-phalangeal joints. The cause is often multifactorial and includes small muscle wasting as a result of diabetic peripheral neuropathy. Previous trauma or surgery can also lead to the development of claw toes. Foot shape deformity may be secondary to factors other than joint restriction. Charcot deformities, nail abnormalities, peripheral oedema and deformities secondary to surgical procedures all increase the risk of foot ulceration.

Ingrowing toenails are a common affliction. Ulceration can develop when the nail penetrates tissue as a result of secondary trauma and infections are common here. The ingrowing toenail is caused by excessive convexity of the nail plate or poor nail care. In diabetic peripheral neuropathy, thickening of the nail and abnormal nail shape can occur, leading to ulceration beneath the nail. Occasionally nail atrophy can also develop. This is often seen where there is nail ischaemia and can also increase the risk of ulceration and infection at the edge of the nail.

Peripheral oedema is frequently found in patients with diabetes, particularly in the elderly. It may exist as a marker of congestive cardiac failure, which is more commonly seen in patients with diabetes. It may also occur in nephrotic syndrome and in situations of malnourishment or where there is organ failure. Oedema is found in patients with severe diabetic neuropathy who have no cardiac disease or other obvious underlying cause.[6] This form of oedema is likely to be secondary to a reduction of sympathetic tone in peripheral vasculature.[7] Changes in blood flow occur as a result of increased vasodilatation and arterio-venous shunting. The resultant increase in venous pressure is worsened by prolonged periods of standing. Ultimately this leads to the development of peripheral oedema.

Oedema is a significant risk factor for the development of foot ulceration, but may also delay recovery from pre-existing foot ulceration. It results in a tighter shoe fit and therefore increases the pressure effects of ill-fitting shoes.

Previous foot surgery is a risk factor for foot ulceration since it may alter pressure distribution significantly. Digital (ray) amputation is the commonest procedure carried out for digital gangrene, a complication that occurs as a result of neuropathic or neuroischaemic damage to a toe. The amputation is often curative but affects the biomechanics of the foot, which leads to increased pressure under the metatarsal heads, increasing the risk of further ulceration.

Neuropathy

Diabetes may affect both central and peripheral nerves. It can affect single or multiple nerves, sensory, motor or autonomic nerves. The commonest risk factor for the development of foot ulceration, however, is chronic sensorimotor neuropathy. This may occur with or without symptoms (painless or painful) and can be seen in the presence or absence of pedal foot pulses (neuropathic or neuroischaemic foot). The prevalence of chronic sensorimotor neuropathy may approach 30 per cent in the UK diabetic population.[8,9] Its prevalence increases with age and duration of diabetes. Its importance here is the magnifying effect it has on the risk of developing diabetic foot ulceration.

Diabetic peripheral neuropathy is predominantly sensory and its distribution is usually symmetrical, with a predilection for the feet. Symptoms are discussed later in the section on neuropathic pain. Early clinical signs include decreased vibration sense, absent ankle reflexes and muscle weakness/wasting. There are many different methods for evaluating and scoring signs of diabetic neuropathy. The classical tools used are tendon hammer, pin, cotton wool swab and a 128 Hz tuning fork. These allow an assessment of reflexes, pain, light touch, vibration and temperature sensation. A validated technique for assessing pressure sensation is the application of a 10 g monofilament to the skin.[8] The National Institute for Clinical Excellence (NICE)[10] recommends the use of a calibrated tuning fork or a 10 g monofilament for assessing sensation. The neurothesiometer is an alternative validated device used to deliver vibrations of varying amplitude. This enables the calculation of a vibration perception threshold.

These methods are all designed to detect those patients at high risk of foot ulceration. Peripheral neuropathy in the foot is initially characterized by small fibre changes – a loss of pain and heat sensation. Later, a mixed fibre neuropathy develops, with small and large myelinated nerve fibres affected. There is then an additional loss of touch, vibration and proprioception sense. This can then lead to weakness and wasting of the intrinsic foot muscles with subsequent deformities of the toes, as described earlier. Secondarily, on weight bearing there will be abnormal pressure distribution and an ill-fitting effect in previously well-fitting footwear may be created. Dryness and fissuring of skin is a frequent feature of diabetic neuropathy, probably as an effect of reduced sweating related to impaired autonomic function. Cracks in the skin provide an entry site for secondary infection.

As discussed previously, foot ulceration predominantly occurs in areas of high pressure.[11] There is good evidence that foot pressures in diabetic patients with peripheral neuropathy are greater than those in those diabetic patients without neuropathy. In addition, these higher pressures are highly predictive of subsequent foot ulceration.[12] Increased weight and foot deformities will exacerbate the risk associated with these increased pressures.

The characteristic complication of the neuropathic foot is the neuropathic ulcer. This is positioned most commonly on the tip of a toe or underneath a metatarsal head. It can also be found on the dorsum of the toe, between toes or underneath the heel. Its appearance is typically 'punched out'. The lesion is often circular, particularly on the sole of the foot, and has surrounding callus formation. It is typically painless but may penetrate to involve deeper tissues, including bone.

Neuropathic ulceration occurs primarily because of a reduction in pain sensation. Loss of pain awareness enables the development and progression of foot lesions to proceed unchecked. The common triggers for the development of foot ulceration include callus formation, direct trauma, excessive heat, chemical trauma and local infection. Neglected callus formation can occur as a result of increased vertical and shear forces beneath the metatarsal heads or excessive friction at the tips of the toes as a result of walking and recurrent trauma of toe against footwear. Repetitive friction or pressure leads to cell damage, microscopic haemorrhage and callus formation. Tissue damage and necrosis beneath the callus leads to the development of small cavities that can fill with serous fluid and erupt onto the surface of the foot as an ulcer.

Ulceration may also develop from more direct trauma such as treading on sharp objects or from debris or irregular surfaces within footwear. Some foot ulcers originate from direct heat trauma. Typical causes include placing feet directly in front of fires and radiators, bathing feet in excessively hot water or placing them against hot water bottles. Loss of pain awareness prevents the sufferer moving his feet away from these stimuli, and direct damage to epithelium then occurs. Chemical burns can similarly occur from using solutions that contain salicylic acid, which is commonly used for treating warts and corns.

Fungal infections are more common in those with diabetes and occur commonly in the inter-digital spaces. This can lead to cracks and breaches in the skin. Secondary infection and ulceration may ensue.

Other factors contributing to the development of neuropathic ulceration include autonomic and motor neuropathy. Autonomic neuropathy leads to dryness of the skin. This can lead to cracks that may provide a portal for infection. It can also lead to arterio-venous shunting, which may affect the perfusion of skin and bone. Motor neuropathy contributes to the paralysis of small muscles in the feet, which in turn may exacerbate structural abnormalities. The classical example of this is clawing of the toes, which leads to prominent metatarsal heads and accompanying high-pressure zones.

Secondary infection frequently contributes to the persistence and worsening of foot ulceration. Typically the organisms involved are the local skin commensals staphylococci and streptococci. These secrete necrotizing toxins and other enzymes that act directly on local small blood vessels to spread infection and cause local thromboses. Spreading cellulitis can develop in surrounding skin or in deeper tissues. A range of tissues including tendons, joints and bones can also become infected. Bacteria and toxins may invade systemically to cause a bacteraemia.

A wide spectrum of bacteria may contribute to persisting infection. These include anaerobic organisms, Gram-negative bacilli and cocci in addition to gas-forming organisms including *Clostridia, E. coli* and *Bacteroides*.

Other complications of infection include local necrosis and gangrene. These can result from damage to microcirculation even when major foot pulses are present.

Impairment of blood supply

Diabetes is partly characterized by its effects on macro- and microcirculation. The circulatory disease of the leg seen in diabetes is different from that of the non-diabetic. The involvement, however, is quite variable. There may be diffuse atherosclerotic changes, patchy distribution or markedly distal distribution of disease.[13,14] Although small vessel disease can lead to impaired local blood supply in diabetes, the absence of palpable peripheral pulses is the typical finding and signifies the potential presence of large vessel disease.

Macrovascular disease in the diabetic leg can occur at the iliac, femoral, popliteal and tibial regions. Those with diabetes have a higher incidence of disease in the arteries distal to the popliteal and have more diffuse vessel involvement. Atherosclerosis tends to be 'multisegmental' rather than involving a single region of arterial wall.[15]

Arterial calcification is commonly observed in radiographs of diabetic feet and hands. This is due to calcification of the media in muscular arteries. Its importance in determining blood flow is not clear, but its effects are probably not significant.[16] However, atherosclerotic disease may appear more commonly in calcified vessels.[17]

Damage to small blood vessels in the feet of diabetic individuals leads to capillary leakage of albumin.[18] Other findings on microscopic examination include obliterative lesions of arterioles and capillaries with basement membrane thickening and endothelial proliferation, but the importance of these findings in determining circulation is not known.

Intermittent claudication and rest pain may be presenting symptoms of major vessel disease. On examination of the diabetic foot the absence of pedal and posterior tibial pulses is an important finding since it indicates the presence of macrovascular disease. Ulceration is a common feature of the neuro-ischaemic foot. Its appearance is different from that of the neuropathic ulcer. Callus is not usually present. Typically there is an area of necrosis surrounded by a rim of erythema. The typical sites of ulceration are the great toe, the medial surface of the first metatarsal head and the heel. Unlike neuropathic ulceration it is frequently painful.

Minor trauma is often the precipitating factor for tissue damage in the ischaemic foot. Simple trauma includes pressure from ill-fitting shoes or even tight socks. Injuries may originate from the cutting of toenails or thermal and chemical injuries outlined previously. If these injuries are ignored, secondary infection commonly occurs. In the ischaemic foot there is frequently blockage of the metatarsal arteries[14] and this reduces communication between plantar and dorsal arterial arches. This lack of collateral circulation can be devastating since bacteria may produce toxins that cause direct damage to local blood vessels. These can lead to obliteration of local arterial blood supply, a problem that is then compounded by the absence of collateral flow.

Management of diabetic foot ulceration

There are common principles that underpin the management of both neuropathic and neuro-ischaemic foot ulceration. These include local medical and surgical treatments, infection control and pressure reduction. The role of arterial surgery is restricted to those with ischaemic disease. It is probably simplest to consider the management of these two forms of foot ulceration separately.

Neuropathic ulceration

Reduction of weight bearing

In the initial stages of acute foot ulceration it is important to reduce weight-bearing. This is essential to promote healing. It can most easily be achieved with bed rest, although this is not generally advised or welcomed by patients. Prolonged immobilization should be avoided since this may lead to thrombo-embolic and other complications.

Although bed rest will remove forces that relate to weight-bearing, care should be taken to prevent pressure on the heels. Foam wedge heel supports are a simple form of protection, but pressure-believing boots and mattresses (e.g. Repose type) are preferable.

Casting techniques offer an alternative to bed rest since they allow the patient to retain mobility. The traditional cast is the total contact plaster cast with simple padding. This can be used for a short period to equalize pressure forces in the affected foot. Removable casts such as the Scotch cast boot are increasingly being used. Additional appliances are available for the reduction of weight-bearing forces. Removable cast walkers such as the Aircast pneumatic diabetic walking boot have superceded the use of scotch cast boots in some centres. Special footwear can be fashioned from casts of the patient's foot. Pressure can also be reduced with insoles made from polyethylene foam that are moulded to the plantar surface of the foot. These insoles can be combined with a layer of tougher rubber to prevent compression. Padded socks have also been used to reduce pressure load.

When using moulded insoles it is important that shoes have more depth to prevent compression or abrasion of the foot. In addition, uppers should be flexible in order to respond to toe pressure.[19] Heels should be stable and the fore-foot area of the shoe wide and square. Lace-ups are essential to prevent foot slippage and resultant trauma to the end of toes. Shoes will need to be customized individually (bespoke) where foot deformity is present and soles should be altered when cushioned insoles do not provide protection. For an ulcer situated beneath a metatarsal head, a common adjustment includes a metatarsal bar which is placed proximal to the metatarsal heads. A rocker sole can be useful for ulcers beneath the first toe since it shifts the pressure load to the mid-foot.

Local treatment

A foot ulcer is surrounded by callus and this needs to be surgically removed. This has the effect of reducing local pressure, allowing effective drainage of the wound, enabling re-epithelialization of the ulcer edges. This should result in an improved rate of healing. An expert in this procedure, usually a specialist podiatrist, should remove the callus. The blade of a scalpel is used to pare away the callus so that the base of the ulcer is fully exposed. The wound and the surrounding skin should then be cleaned with a sterile saline solution. The ulcer should be covered with a clean non-adhesive dressing. This procedure will need to be repeated frequently until the ulcer is healed. There is evidence that growth factor-containing gels and membranes may improve the healing rate of diabetic foot ulceration, but the cost may be prohibitive and their use may be restricted to difficult non-healing ulcers.[20]

High-dose, broad-spectrum antibiotic therapy is advocated.[21] There are a number of reasons for this. Tissue penetration may be poor and low doses of antibiotic may lead to inadequate levels within the target tissue. There is a wide spectrum of organisms implicated in the development of an infected foot ulcer, many of which may be opportunistic skin commensals. Typical organisms include staphylococci, streptococci, Gram-negative bacteria and anaerobes.

Oral antibiotic therapy may be used in the first instance. Co-amoxiclav, in the form of Augmentin, 625 mg three times daily for a period of 2 weeks is our locally recommended treatment regime. There are different recommendations in other heath localities. Therapy choice is hampered by the absence of a good evidence base. This is due to a lack of adequate clinical trials.

In the presence of spreading cellulitis, surrounding erythema or skin discolouration, the use of antibiotics is indicated urgently. A typical intravenous antibiotic regimen would be cefuroxime, 1.5 mg three times daily, and metronidazole, 1 g three times daily. The choice of intravenous agent will depend upon whether there is bone involvement and whether there has been recent hospitalization with the concurrent increased risk of methicillin-resistant *Staphylococcus aureus* (MRSA). In this case intravenous Vancomycin may be added.

It is imperative that collections of pus and abscess cavities are drained surgically. Necrotic tissue in a neuropathic foot should also be removed surgically. Typically, gangrene in a digit requires a ray amputation – the surgical removal of the affected phalanx and metatarsal head.[22] This is a well-established and effective treatment.

Neuro-ischaemic ulceration

The management of this condition incorporates a range of therapeutic options that are similar to those used in the treatment of neuropathic ulceration. Surgical management is required for the excision of necrotic tissue and to improve blood supply to the affected area.

Unlike neuropathic ulceration, ischaemic ulceration is frequently painful. This can sometimes be successfully treated with simple or codeine-based therapy, but frequently only responds to regular opioid analgesia. Swabs should be taken for bacterial culture from the ulcer site. Ulcers should be cleaned with a sterile saline solution. Only sterile, non-adherent dressings should be applied to the cleansed wound.

Antibiotic therapy is necessary for infected ulcers. High-dose, broad-spectrum agents should be used pending further information about organism sensitivities from wound swab cultures. Infected ulcers that exhibit more than a surrounding rim of erythema or which penetrate deeply require intravenous antibiotic therapy.

Appropriate footwear may include require shoes of extra depth to avoid friction effects.

In the deformed foot a bespoke shoe may be required. All necrotic tissue contained within an ischaemic ulcer needs to be surgically excised by an advanced podiatrist or an appropriately trained surgeon. If ulcers are situated beneath the nail (sub-ungual), the nail may need to be cut back or excised to allow drainage of the ulcer. Any focal collection of pus (abscess) also requires surgical drainage.

In patients with neuro-ischaemic ulceration consideration should be given to further investigation with a view to surgical therapy. Unfortunately peripheral vascular disease frequently co-exists with significant cardiovascular or cerebro-vascular disease. This may render an individual patient unsuitable for a surgical procedure and needs to be assessed on an individual basis.

The increased emphasis on limb salvage and the development of new techniques of re-vascularization has led to a reduction in the frequency of major amputation in patients with diabetic foot ulceration. This has direct financial benefits given that successful re-vascularization has been associated with improved mobility[23] and costs less than amputation.[24]

The conventional non-invasive technique for identifying limb ischaemia is Doppler ultrasound. This technique assesses the velocity of blood flow and the pressure index within lower limb arteries. This process can, however, be unreliable in patients with significant arterial wall calcification – a common finding in diabetes. This can now be complemented by Duplex ultrasound, which demonstrates in more detail the anatomy and function of vessels.

Improvements in arteriography, and in particular digital subtraction arteriography, have enabled even better views of diseased distal limb vessels. The detection and characterization of limb ischaemia in those with diabetes has been significantly enhanced by these modern vascular imaging techniques.

There have also been advances in percutaneous angioplasty techniques. Angioplasty has become established in the treatment of diabetic peripheral vascular disease. Modern catheter techniques allow balloons that incorporate guide wires to be passed into distal vessels to dilate strictures. As a technique angioplasty is minimally invasive and associated with a low risk of complications and a short duration of hospital stay.

Percutaneous catheterization also allows for the local introduction of thrombolytic therapy although this requires further studies.

Arterial bypass therapy has traditionally been fraught with difficulty in patients with peripheral vascular disease and diabetes because of the distal and diffuse nature of the atherosclerotic disease. However, in carefully selected patients, limb salvage and graft patency are improved in distal bypass grafts to both the dorsalis pedis and posterior tibial arteries.[25,26] Although this form of surgery may require repeat surgical procedures, the typical cost remains less than that of major amputation.[24]

Arterial reconstruction has become more commonplace as our understanding of the pattern of vascular disease in diabetes has improved. Pre-operative imaging techniques have given vascular surgeons a greater understanding and knowledge of the distribution of vascular disease in given individuals. In addition, the use of autologous vein grafts rather than prosthetic grafts has increased patency and limb salvage rates.[25] The re-vascularization of feet via distal arterial reconstruction appears to provide good capillary perfusion despite the presence of diabetes.[27]

3.3   Charcot Foot

In 1868, Charcot first described the neuropathic joint degeneration that occurs in diseases where loss of sensation predominates. In the past Charcot disease has been considered rare in diabetes, but it may be more common than previously understood and may also be under-diagnosed in its acute presentation.[28]

The mechanism of the bone damage associated with Charcot disease appears to be an increase in blood flow that may be secondary to the loss of sympathetic nerve supply associated with neuropathic disease. This causes increased osteoclast activity within bone and bone turnover is increased, leading to increased bone fragility. Susceptible bone becomes more prone to damage and fracture from minor trauma and there is subsequent destruction of bony architecture. This problem is compounded by the inevitable presence of peripheral sensory neuropathy that also alters the natural gait pattern. There is also a reduced range of motion of the joints, caused by glycosylation of connective tissue. These factors lead to greater strain on the foot and bones within, worsening the destructive bone disease. If locomotion continues with less than optimal foot function then the plantar fascia may also become damaged. The presence of diabetic neuropathy may result in these changes being asymptomatic. This may delay individuals from seeking corrective treatment.

Acute Charcot foot

Acute Charcot foot (neuro-arthropathy) is a progressive but self-limiting condition. It occurs in those with peripheral neuropathy and a good vascular supply. It can occur in patients with both type 1 and type 2 diabetes.

The patient frequently presents with a hot, swollen foot that may be painful. Complaints may include noises 'like bones cracking' or odd, uncomfortable sensations 'like stones rubbing against each other inside my feet'. The typical affected sites are the tarsal–metatarsal region or the metatarso-phalangeal joints. Peripheral pulses are invariably present and peripheral neuropathy is evident clinically. If only one foot is affected there may be a considerable temperature differential between the two. Most patients remain mobile and usually walk into the consulting room. In many cases trauma may be the trigger for the development of Charcot foot. However this is not universal and in the patient who is profoundly neuropathic the trauma may, of course, pass unnoticed. The differential diagnoses for acute Charcot disease include cellulitis, gout and deep vein thrombosis. Radiographic imaging and isotope bone scans can assist in diagnosis, but this can still prove difficult in the early stages.

As the disease progresses, the structure of the foot is destroyed. Joint dislocations and fractures occur. These are often in the mid-foot, leading to the collapse of the arch. This can result in a rocker-bottom deformity due to displacement and subluxation of the tarsus or medial convexity due to the talo-navicular joint or tarso-metatarsal dislocation.

The foot should be reviewed and treated until the swelling has subsided and temperature has returned to normal. During this period, patients will need support and reassurance. The condition takes a variable amount of time to resolve and this can cause significant anxiety.

The key to treatment, and long-term preservation of the limb, is immobilization. This will prevent further joint damage and should be recommended immediately. Continued walking will inevitably lead to ulceration and more damage.

Options for immobilization include crutches, wheelchair, total contact cast and replaceable cast walker. These allow patients to mobilize safely and usually without pain. Immobilization is recommended for a period of 2–3 months, but can be as long as a year, depending upon the activity of the disease.

Bisphosphonates such as pamidronate may be administered by intravenous infusion. These can reduce swelling, pain and redness.[29] They work by reducing osteoclast activity during the acute phase of Charcot disease.

When the acute phase has resolved, the foot should be reviewed and future care must be planned. The patient should be considered at high risk for ulceration. If deformity is minimal, a foot protection team should review the patient and ongoing foot support provided. If there is deformity that makes it difficult to obtain appropriate footwear (see below) or if weight bearing is considered dangerous or likely to cause ulceration, then an orthotic referral for alternative footwear provision is necessary. In some cases more invasive management may be required. An orthopaedic opinion for consideration of reconstructive surgery may be useful in helping to restore normal foot shape.

Some patients may present with both foot ulceration and acute Charcot foot simultaneously. In this situation management should be offered for both conditions through appropriately developed care pathways.

Chronic Charcot foot

Charcot disease may present with the disabling complications more frequently than the acute features. Deformity is a frequent finding and will predispose the affected foot to ulceration and infection. Management needs to reflect this common presentation and should include preventative aspects of foot ulcer management together with a treatment plan to minimize the effects of the deformity.

Minor deformity may be managed in normal footwear with the addition of insoles or orthoses. Bespoke footwear and insoles may be required and allow the patient to walk without risking trauma and secondary ulceration.

Surgery can transform a rocker bottom foot to a planti-grade foot. This allows for safe weight-bearing. The feet of these patients will remain at high risk; they will need to be maintained and supported by podiatrists in a foot protection team (Figure 3.1).

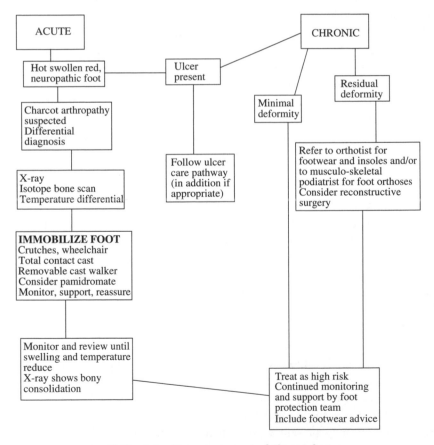

Figure 3.1 The management of Charcot foot

3.4   Nerve Damage and Painful Diabetic Neuropathy

Terminology

There are many different descriptive terms used in the management of diabetic neuropathy and health care professionals can easily become confused. We have described below a number of terms and their explanations in an attempt to demystify them.

- *Neuropathy* – 'neuro' meaning nerve, 'pathy' meaning damage, therefore 'damaged nerve'.

- *Mononeuropathy* – damage to one nerve. Peripheral or cranial mononeuropathies are fairly commonplace. They may be spontaneous or secondary to entrapment or external pressure. Carpal tunnel syndrome can occur in up to 30 per cent of patients with diabetes,[30] with symptoms occurring in 10 per cent. Patients complain of pain in the hands or forearm, typically worse at night and early morning. Nerve conduction studies should be used to confirm the diagnosis. Although overnight wrist supports may be helpful in alleviating symptoms, definitive treatment requires surgical decompression. Entrapment of the common peroneal nerve of the thigh is seen more commonly in patients with diabetes. This can give pain and parasthesia in the outer third of the thigh.
  Spontaneous neuropathy occurs in the common peroneal nerve and leads to foot drop. Full recovery is not usual and there is no definitive therapy. The commonest cranial nerves affected are the third and sixth. In third nerve palsy the patient may complain of pain in the orbital region or frontal headache. There is typically ptosis and ophthalmoplegia, although the papillary reflexes are usually spared. Recovery usual occurs within 3 months. CT or MRI scanning is required in cranial nerve palsies to exclude raised pressure secondary to local aneurysm formation or a space occupying brain lesion. Axillary, ulnar and other nerves can be damaged by external pressure – occasionally wrist drop can occur in patients unconscious from hypoglycaemia or following an alcohol binge.

- *Polyneuropathy* – where more than one individual nerve is affected or damaged.

- *Distal symmetrical polyneuropathy* – sometimes referred to as 'diabetic neuropathy', 'sensory neuropathy' or 'chronic distal sensorimotor polyneuropathy', this is the characteristic neurological impairment in diabetes where foot sensation is predominantly affected. There is a symmetrical loss of light touch, pinprick, vibration and temperature perception in distal limbs. The physiology is discussed in more detail later.

- *Sensory ataxia* – a loss of proprioception, the ability to distinguish joint position. This results in a loss of balance and a resultant high incidence of falls.

- *Neuritis* – acute nerve inflammation.

- *Insulin neuritis* – an acute painful neuropathy relating to a rapid alteration of glycaemic control. Symptoms include burning sensations, allodynia (see pain descriptors), nocturnal exacerbation and numbness. Sensory loss is usually mild or absent with no motor involvement. There is little or no abnormality in nerve conduction studies and usually a complete resolution of symptoms within 12 months. Depressive symptoms are common.

- *Acute painful neuropathy of poor glycaemic control* – this condition presents in patients with both type 1 and type 2 diabetes. It occurs in the presence of poor glycaemic control. There is often associated weight loss that improves with the resolution of symptoms. Pain is worse at night but there is typically persistent 'background ' pain. Ellenberg coined the phrase 'neuropathic cachexia' to describe the symptoms of neuropathic pain, poor glycaemic control and weight loss. On examination sensory loss is typically mild or even absent, ankle jerks may be absent and nerve conduction tests are usually normal or mildly abnormal. The temperature discrimination threshold is affected (small fibres) more commonly than the vibration perception threshold (large fibre involvement). There is a complete resolution within 12 months and weight gain is usual with continued improvement in glycaemic control and with the use of insulin.

- *Diabetic amyotrophy* – also termed 'proximal motor neuropathy' (PMN), 'femoral neuropathy' or 'symmetrical proximal lower limb motor neuropathy'. This occurs in type 1 and type 2 diabetes (typically in patients aged less than 50 years). Patients complain of severe pain deep in the thigh or burning pain extending below the knee. Pain is usually continuous and is frequently associated with insomnia and depression. Patients may experience difficulty in rising out of chairs, climbing stairs etc. There may be associated weight loss and this raises the possibility of occult malignancy. Symptoms may begin unilaterally or bilaterally. An unaffected side usually becomes involved within a few weeks. On examination there is profound wasting of the quadriceps muscles with marked weakness. Hip flexor and thigh abductor muscles can be affected. Glutei and hamstring muscles may also be involved. The knee jerk is usually absent or reduced. There may be localized sensory loss over thigh. In this condition it is important to exclude other causes of proximal muscle wasting. These include nerve root and cauda equina lesions, occult malignancy and polymyositis. Investigations should include an erythrocyte sedimentation rate (ESR), radiographic imaging of lumbar spine and chest, and abdominal ultrasound where indicated. Electrophysiological studies may demonstrate increased femoral nerve latency and active denervation of affected muscles. Occasionally an MRI of the lumbo-sacral spine may be required to exclude focal nerve root entrapment. The pain usually settles within three months. At 2 years the knee jerk reflex has returned in 50 per cent of affected patients. Management of this condition is essentially supportive. Sufferers should be informed that it is likely to resolve. There is controversy as to whether the use of insulin offers additional benefit, but it should be prescribed in patients with poor control despite oral therapy. Physiotherapy aimed at strengthening the quadriceps muscles may be helpful.

- *Truncal radiculopathy or thoraco-abdominal neuropathy* – this condition is rare. Sufferers typically present with acute asymmetrical pain with patchy sensory loss over the thorax and/or abdomen. The onset is rapid but recovery occurs within 3–12 months. There may be associated weight loss and aching, burning or sharp pain. Other causes of nerve root compression need to be excluded.

- *Autonomic neuropathy* – this is damage to sympathetic and parasympathetic nervous systems. This is found, to some extent, in 30 per cent of patients with diabetes. The most common symptom is erectile dysfunction. Other problems include gastrointestinal dysfunction (delayed gastric emptying, nausea, vomiting, dysphagia, diarrhoea/constipation) and bladder dysfunction (urinary retention/overflow incontinence). Postural hypotension can lead to dizziness and syncope. Tachycardia or sinus arrythmias can be difficult to manage perioperatively. Absent or excessive (gustatory) sweating can also occur. Dryness of the feet can cause cracks in the skin and provide portals for infection.

Chronic peripheral sensorimotor neuropathy

This is present in up to 60 per cent of patients with diabetes, although abnormalities on history and examination are found in only 20 per cent.[31] The condition becomes increasingly common with increasing duration of diabetes. There is a link between poor glycaemic control.[32] and the development of diabetic peripheral neuropathy in both type 1 and type 2 diabetes. The mechanism is not fully understood but there are clear links with the impairment of blood supply to myelinated and unmyelinated nerve fibres. Nerve damage may be sporadic and non-selective with a predilection therefore for the longest nerves, principally those supplying the feet, and to a lesser extent the hands. Unlike nociceptive pain (see later descriptors) neurological pain occurs when there are chemical and anatomical changes in nerve function. Pain can be a presenting feature in patients newly diagnosed with diabetes.[33,35]

Patients with this condition are at increased risk of developing retinopathy and nephropathy. Unlike these microvascular complications, however, the evidence does not suggest that the aetiological factor is non-enzymatic glycosylation of structural proteins.

Sensorimotor neuropathy is so common that it is tempting to forget that there are other causes of peripheral neuropathy. These include alcohol, B_{12} and other vitamin deficiencies, drug treatment and malignancy.

Causes of peripheral neuropathy

- *Metabolic* – diabetes, uraemia, amyloidosis, myxoedema and porphyria.

- *Nutritional* – B_{12}, B_6, nicotinic acid or thiamine deficiencies.

- *Drug/chemical* – nitrofurantoin, vincristine, chloambucil, isoniazid, phenytoin.

- *Neoplasia* – brochogenic carcinoma, malignant lymphoma.

- *Infection* – Guillain–Barré syndrome, leprosy.

- *Genetic* – Charcot–Marie–Tooth syndrome.

- *Organ failure* – renal and hepatic failure.

Assessment of peripheral neuropathy

Tools used for the assessment and detection of neuropathy can be simple. As mentioned previously, techniques include the assessment of ankle/knee reflexes using a tendon hammer, assessment of vibration perception with the use of a 128 Hz tuning fork, light touch/pressure sensation using a cotton wool swab[34] or 10 g monofilament and pain sensation using the 'Neurotip' or a neurological pin. It is important that health areas standardize tools used to assess nerve function. A 10 g monofilament should be used to assess fine touch.[10,35] These can form part of a 'baseline foot assessment tool' that combines aspects of history and examination to identify those patients at high risk of developing foot ulceration.[36] Patients who score as 'high risk' as a result of sensory loss in combination with other risk findings should receive increased monitoring education advice and support from an advanced podiatry team.

Neuropathy – screening techniques and investigation

Monofilament testing

A 10 g 'monofilament' developed from a set of nylon filaments is used to assess cutaneous sensation (large nerve fibre function). It should be used at multiple sites on the dorsum of the foot. Buckling of the filament above a threshold allows a constant pressure to be applied.[35]

Vibration measurement

A 128 Hz tuning fork detects core vibration sensation (large fibre). Sites tested should include the pulp of the great toe and bony prominence of the medial malleolus.

Biothesiometer

This is a hand-held electronic device containing a vibrating probe. The voltage is altered and this affects the vibration amplitude of the probe. The amplitude is increased until the patient can feel the vibration. This creates a 'vibration perception threshold' (VPT) for each individual. The VPT provides a quantitative assessment of neuropathy.

Computer-added sensory evaluator (CASE IV)

This is one of a number of systems used to detect loss of temperature sensation (small myelinated and unmyelinated fibres transmit cold and warmth, respectively). These instruments are not currently in routine clinical use since testing is frequently lengthy and results are variable.

Foot pain – descriptive terms

- *Neuropathic pain* – this is pain caused by a primary lesion or dysfunction of the nervous system (International Association of the Study of Pain, IASP).

- *Nociceptive pain* – this is pain that occurs when usual nerve function and pain pathways are in working order. It warns the individual of actual or potential tissue damage, e.g. pain resulting from stepping on a drawing pin.

- *Chronic pain* – this is described as pain that lasts for more than 3 months (IASP). Clinical trials frequently prefer to define it as painful symptoms lasting for 12 months or more.

- *Metatarsalgia* – this is pain that occurs beneath the metatarsal heads of the forefoot. A common descriptive term used by patients with this condition is 'like walking on marbles'.

- *Hyperaesthesia* – this is a heightened awareness of sensations or increased sensitivity to stimulation, e.g. brushing or stroking of the skin.

- *Hypoaesthesia* – this is a decreased sensitivity to stimulation.

- *Hyperpathia* – this is a pain syndrome characterized by abnormally painful reactions to stimuli.

- *Analgesia* – this is the absence of pain to stimuli that would normally be painful.

- *Hypoalgesia* – this is diminished pain in response to normally painful stimuli.

- *Hyperalgesia* – this is an increased response to a stimuli that is not normally painful.

- *Allodynia* – this is the alteration of normal sensation into a painful or unpleasant sensation or pain due to a stimulus that does not usually provoke pain (IASP).

- *Paraesthesiae* – this is a difficult sensation to describe. 'Pins and needles' is an accurate if unscientific descriptor. It is an important discriminator between 'neuropathic pain' and the 'rest pain' of peripheral ischeamia.

Risk factors for the development of painful diabetic neurpathy

- Increased age.

- Poor glycaemic control.

- Increased duration of diabetes.

- Smoking.

- Other microvascular complications – established complications such as nephropathy or retinopathy.

- Abnormal lipid metabolism – low levels of high-density lipoprotein (HDL).

Assessment of foot pain

It is essential when assessing a patient with foot pain to take a detailed history. This should include detailed information about the type, frequency and nature of the pain, precipitating and alleviating factors and other associated symptoms.[37] A detailed past medical and medication history should be sought. There should be specific questioning about the presence of back pain and bowel/bladder function. It is essential to rule out other causes of foot/leg pain and the other causes of peripheral neuropathy. The pain may be severe and it is important to allow the patient to express their feelings and for the listener to be empathetic. An assessment of the impact of symptoms should be made.

A full physical examination should be carried out. This should include a clinical neurological assessment. Pain is subjective and it may be important to identify tools that enable symptoms to be quantified.[35,38] Pain questionnaires are widely used to assist in the detection and measurement of severity of pain and in the evaluation of treatment. Common questionnaires and tools in use include the following:

- *Visual analogue scale* (VAS)[38] – patients quantify their pain on a scale of 0 (no pain) to 10 (worst pain ever). This gives a quantitative assessment of the pain severity.

- *McGill pain questionaire*[39] – this questionnaire is able to quantify the quality and severity of pain using four categories: sensory, affective, evaluative and miscellaneous. Descriptive terms are ranked by intensity.

- *DYCKS neuropathic staging*[38,39] – this takes into account the severity of pain but also grades the impact of 'numbness' and ataxia. The grading takes into account the impact on lifestyle', e.g. attending a physician for pain relief, effects on work and recreational activities and need for medication.

- *LANNS neuropathic pain scale*[34] – this pain questionnaire takes into account functional problems as well as pain perception.

Management of neuropathic pain

There are a variety of treatments available for the management of neuropathic pain. However, success in alleviating all pain is unrealistic for many. Frequently the goal is an improved quality of life, improved sleep and a *reduction* in pain. A 50 per cent reduction in pain severity may be a realistic and adequate goal. The response to differing treatments will vary markedly between individuals.

Improvement in glycaemic control may help to prevent the development and progression of neuropathic pain, and it is important to target a lowering of blood glucose in those patients who have poor control. Painful neuropathic symptoms can, however, worsen acutely in the context of both sudden deterioration and sudden improvement in glycaemic control. The aim should therefore be a gradual improvement. Patients with type 2 diabetes and poor glucose control despite maximal oral hypoglycaemic agents should be commenced on insulin therapy.

Neuropathic pain is usually a self-limiting condition but symptoms can last for many years. It is important to inform sufferers about the cause and natural history of the condition. This information should include a careful explanation of different treatments, their effectiveness, potential side-effects and likely improvements. It is essential that support networks are put in place for patients. We have found that an education group involving patients, those that care for them and interested health care professionals is one way of achieving this. This has the benefit of providing peer support and also empowering patients with persisting pain to seek further treatment and support. The authors have come to realize the importance of involving patients in decision-making.

It is common for patients to require a number of different treatments, either alone or in combination. It is vital that treatment is continuously monitored and adjusted in order to maximize the beneficial effects. This may prove difficult in a busy specialty outpatient setting but can be achieved more easily by involving patients in their management through self-titration of drug therapy and agreed care protocols. By establishing for patients an easy point of contact with an interested health care professional, this benefit is further enhanced.

Medical therapies

We recommend the use of an algorithm to standardize the management of neuropathic pain so that individual patients can receive benefit from all available treatments in an order that is most appropriate for achieving resolution of symptoms and improvement in quality of life (Figure 3.2).

Simple painkillers are rarely effective and their use should not be prolonged unless there is a rapid response to treatment.

Topical agents

Capsaicin cream (0.075 per cent) is derived from the chilli pepper. This is applied three to four times daily to symptomatic areas of the foot. It is believed to work through depletion of substance P from nerve terminals.

The use of this agent should be reserved for superficial discomfort and pain (burning, tingling etc.). Symptoms (particularly 'burning') may worsen for a period of 2–4 weeks following its initial use. The full benefit of this treatment may not be realized for 6 weeks. It is essential that patients are well educated in the use of this product in order for it to be effective. Hands need to be washed before and immediately after use. Contact with eyes and inflamed or broken skin should be

Diagnosis
Consider reversible causes, e.g.
B_{12} deficiency and alchololism

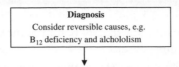

Education and explanation. Outline coping strategies and prognosis
Address poor glycaemic control
Prescribe simple analgesia, e.g. paracetamol one month – early review if distressed
Involve physiotherapist where muscle weakness or reduced mobility exists

Ineffective or partially effective

For superficial pain:
Try capsaicin cream (with detailed explanation of its use and side effects) or an
alternative topical application of Opsite spray.

Ineffective or partially effective

Add or start **tricyclic** drug, i.e. amitriptyline, or imipramine with detailed
explanation of use and side effects
Six week course of maximum tolerated dose involving patients in self-titration of doses

Ineffective or partially effective

Consider withdrawal of other oral therapies and introduce a phased course of
gabapentin or pregabalin

Ineffective or partially effective

Consider use of tramadol as an add-on or subsititute therapy

Ineffective or partially effective

Consider substitution of tricyclics or gabapentin/pregabalin for carbamazepine or
Phenytoin **therapy**

Ineffective or partially effective

Consider mechanical or invasive treatments, i.e. TENS, nerve blocks,
sympathectomy, I.V. lignocaine

Ineffective or partially effective

Revisit coping strategies and psychological/psychiatric disease
Consider complementary therapies
Consider referral to specialist pain management team

Figure 3.2 Treatment options in the management of painful peripheral neuropathy

avoided. It should not be used under tight bandages. The patient should also avoid taking a hot shower or bath immediately before or after applying the cream since this exacerbates the burning sensation.

'*Opsite*' spray is an alternative therapy that is sprayed directly onto the affected area gives some patients dramatic cooling relief of symptoms. This therapy can unfortunately be somewhat messy, leaving a filmy residue on the skin surface that can be difficult to remove.

Oral agents

Tricylcyclic antidepressant medication has, for many years, been a first line systemic therapy that is effective in neuropathic pain. Imipramine has been shown to be beneficial in 60 per cent of symptomatic patients. The initial starting dose is 25–50 mg increased in 25 mg increments every 1–2 weeks to a maximum of 150 mg. Amitriptyline as an alternative treatment with a similar dosing schedule has proved to be similarly effective. Side effects of the tricyclic group include sedation, dry mouth, urinary retention, postural hypotension and exacerbation of glaucoma. Treatment protocols can be drawn up to allow patients to self-titrate increases in the dose of these drugs.

Selective serotonin reuptake inhibitors such as paroxetine, citalopram and sibutramine have been used, but have not proved as effective as the tricyclics. Depression can be a common problem occurring in people with chronic pain and it is thought that the antidepressant effect of these drugs may be the mechanism of action through which some benefit was observed.[31]

Anticonvulsants

Gabapentin (Neurontin) and its more recent successor *pregabalin* (Lyrica) are licensed as oral agents for use in painful neuropathy. The mode of action for these drugs is a blockage of neural transmission of pain pathways at the dorsal horns of the spinal cord. Dose titration for gabapentin is in four stages over a 2 week period. A frequent maintenance dose is 600 mg three times daily. Inadequate dose titration of gabapentin will produce a sub-optimal response. Common side-effects are dizziness and drowsiness.

Pregabalin has a similar mode of action and appears to be as effective in the treatment of neuropathic pain. It may have benefits over its predecessor. Dose titration is simpler and quicker. The drug is taken twice daily. Benefits are seen within a week of therapy and improvements in sleep pattern changes are noticeable. The usual final treatment dose is 300 mg twice daily.

Carbamazepine and *phenytoin* have been used in the treatment of neuropathic pain but side effects are common and these drugs are now used less frequently. Sodium valproate has been used less widely.

The use of *opiate-based therapies* is controversial in the management of any chronic pain. These therapies typically cause a degree of dependence but may be advocated in severe intractable cases. *Tramadol* is a centrally acting opioid deriviative that is less addictive and has been shown to benefit some patients with neuropathic pain. A typical daily dose is 200–400 mg.

Intravenous lignocaine has been shown to benefit some patients with intractable neuropathic pain. It is not extensively used due to the need for close cardiac monitoring. A typical starting dose is 5 mg/kg body weight and it is typically infused over 30–60 min. Symptom relief may last for up to 15 days. After this period some physicians have found that the addition of oral mexilitine following a good response can offer additional benefit.[40]

Ketamine is an anaesthetic drug with good analgesic properties when used in sub-anaesthetic dosage. It is administered intramuscularly and may provide temporary pain relief for individuals with severe neuropathic pain. There is, however, a high incidence of hallucinations and other transient psychotic effects reported with this drug. It is usually only considered for use where close monitoring can be provided within a specialist setting.

Other therapies

Spinal cord stimulation TENS machines may be beneficial for some, particularly in those patients with pain localized to one limb only.

Spinal nerve blocks have been used with mixed success but can be considered after an appropriate anaesthetic assessment from within a pain team.

Complementary therapies

Complementary therapies can be used as an adjunct to conventional therapies. For some individuals they can be useful in reducing the impact of this painful condition on quality of life and daily function.[41]

Complementary therapies for managing chronic pain can be split into three categories: physical treatments, relaxation and mind body techniques, and herbal remedies.

- *Physical approaches* – these include therapeutic massage, chiropractic, reflexology, acupuncture and magnetic therapy. There is emerging evidence of the successful role of the use of acupuncture in treating painful diabetic neuropathy.[41,46] It has been suggested that acupuncture works through stimulating energy flow through painful areas. It is being used increasingly within the pain clinic setting. No untoward side effects have been reported. Magnetic therapy is also an emerging therapy in the UK. It has been employed to treat a variety of medical conditions in Asia, predominantly China. Magnetic insoles are one such application. They are thought to stimulate reflexology points in the foot to assist in symptom reduction. In one large study[42] there were statistically significant reductions in pain, burning, numbness and tingling. Care should be taken if employing this technique. When placed in the shoe the insole can raise the foot and a larger toe box is required. If the insole is not cut to the correct shape, pressure ulcers can also develop on the heel.

- *Relaxation techniques* – relaxation techniques may help some to cope with chronic pain. They can help to reduce stress and anxiety that can exacerbate pain. Available therapies include hypnotherapy, meditation, music therapy, yoga, humour therapy and guided imagery.

- *Herbal medicines and aromatherapy* – these have been used for many centuries to treat pain. Many of today's most potent drug therapies are herbal derivatives and it is important not to underestimate their power when used in conjunction with more orthodox treatments. A registered qualified herbalist should carry out the preparation of any herbal remedy.

Psychological support

When managing the chronic pain of peripheral neuropathy it is important to consider whether psychological support may be required. Depressive symptoms are common in this group.[41] There is a strong association between poor glycaemic control and the prevalence of depression.[43] There is also evidence to link loss of proprioception and balance in diabetic patients with an increased incidence of depression.[43] Unfortunately there is a lack of appropriately trained clinical psychologists and others to deal with the psychological effects of chronic pain in diabetes teams.

For the sufferer the effects of trying to cope with symptoms include:

- apathy and self-imposed social isolation;

- an inability to perform the normal activities of daily living;

- disrupted sleep patterns;

- memory impairment;

- mood swings;

- feelings of isolation, frustration and despair;

- suicidal tendencies. (reproduced from *Diabetic Neuropathy – Under the Spotlight*. Booklet, The Neuropathy Trust, 2002.)

The symptoms of painful diabetic neuropathy may affect family and friends. Sleepless nights caused by neuropathic pain can disturb the household and leave the sufferer weary and irritable. This can affect relationships with partner, family and friends.

Many different agents and techniques have been used to manage this condition. It is important to recognize that different individuals respond to different forms of treatment. Alternative therapies may be found to be effective for a given sufferer.

3.5 The Organization of Foot Care

People with diabetes and those caring for them should be provided with easy access to a multidisciplinary diabetic foot care team. This may take the form of the 'gold-standard' multidisciplinary foot clinic. Alternatively this may be a team of people who work closely together in settings that allow for easy communication and direct access to each other's specialist skills.

There should be an organised programme of foot care that includes:

- continuous education of patients carers and staff;

- identification of patients with feet at high risk;

- provision of measures designed to reduce risk;

- streamlined communication between health care professionals that crosses boundaries of care.

A diabetes foot care team can help to provide appropriate knowledge to each other and to others who provide care outside the group. Skills should be made easily accessible to patients and other health carers. The group should produce and disseminate practical guidelines on the avoidance, identification and management of complications. There should be clear pathways between primary and secondary care.[36,44]

A multidisciplinary diabetic foot care team should incorporate a number of key individuals. From the specialist setting there should be a minimum of one individual representing the following areas: specialist podiatry, specialist orthotics, diabetes nurse specialist, consultant diabetologist, vascular surgeon and orthopaedic surgeon. It may be beneficial to involve wound care/tissue viability nurses, plaster technicians and vascular/diabetes/medical admissions ward nurses. Ideally the group should cross the primary/secondary care boundary and incorporate primary care nurse, physician and podiatrist. There should also be a patient representative.

It is not feasible for all of these individuals to be involved in one multi-disciplinary foot clinic. However crucial leaders of the team should meet regularly to enhance the development of a co-ordinated diabetes foot care service.[45] The multidisciplinary foot care team should act as a focal point and resource for patients and other health care professionals.

The team of people caring for those with diabetes is much larger than these few individuals. Extended team members include the patient carer, reception staff, pharmacist, microbiologist, physiotherapist, occupational therapist, clinical psychologist, pain specialist, radiologist and others.

In order to meet the needs and achieve high standards of care for the person with diabetes there needs to be continuing education for all in addition to effective

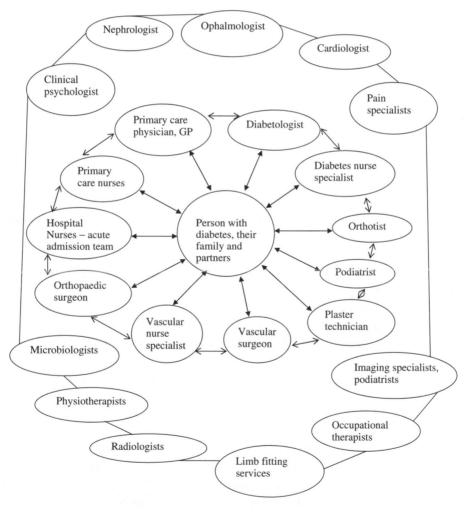

Figure 3.3   The multidisciplinary foot team

communication between all of these individuals. It is the responsibility of the team to ensure that this happens.

Although foot disease is a leading cause of hospital admission and expense,[2] its prevention may increasingly lie in educating patients and staff away from the specialist care setting. We have also therefore helped indicate the links between primary and secondary care to ensure that risk factors are recognized and acted upon and complications are managed effectively (Figure 3.3).

3.6 Conclusion

Care of the diabetic foot requires input before, during and following the development of complications. Prevention of foot ulceration can be optimized by educating patients with diabetes about the use of appropriate footwear and by regular reinforcement of foot-care advice. The annual, thorough inspection of feet is an essential part of a diabetic examination. Standards should be in place to help identify at-risk feet. A baseline foot assessment tool can serve this purpose. In particular the feet of diabetic patients should be carefully examined for the presence of deformities, callus, reduced blood supply and nerve damage.

A good system of foot care should mean that the identification of an at-risk foot triggers the involvement of other health care professionals (orthotist, podiatrist, nurse and doctor) so that the risk of progression to a diseased foot is minimized.

Ulceration of the diabetic foot depends on the presence of neuropathy and/or impaired blood supply. It is particularly likely to occur where high-pressure areas develop. This can be due to the neuropathic process and/or areas of foot deformity. The development of excessive callus is frequently a predictive factor and can break down and lead to secondary ulceration.

Impaired blood supply is due to atherosclerosis involving large vessels of both legs. This is frequently distal and multisegmental, involving tibial and peroneal blood vessels. Areas of pressure that can lead to necrosis compound this reduction in blood supply.

Nerve damage leads to reduction in heat and pain sensation. It also affects blood supply, resulting in diminished sweating. Altered blood flow results in oedema and reduction in bone density. Charcot disease can be a debilitating complication.

Damage to the peripheral nerve fibres can lead to neuropathic pain. This can be a difficult condition to treat. Patients are educated about its cause and the natural history of the condition. They should receive detailed information about treatment options and their likely effectiveness. Systems should be put in place to enable medication to be altered and optimized quickly and effectively.

Optimal care of the diabetic foot is essential and can only be achieved through close collaboration of podiatrist, orthotist, nurse, physician and surgeon. This can most easily be carried out in a dedicated multi-disciplinary foot clinic. Alternatively, there needs to be a system in place that enables easy dialogue and access between these different specialties. The development of an efficient system of care requires the involvement of a dedicated group of individuals representing each specialty. This allows for the development of local care pathways and systems to support the patient with diabetic foot disease. Support networks should transcend any primary/secondary care boundaries.

References

1. Neil HAW, Thompson AV, Thorogood M, Fowler GH, Mann JL. Diabetes in the elderly: the Oxford community diabetes study. *Diabet Med* 1989; **6**: 608–613.
2. Young MJ, Bready JL, Veves A, Boulton AJM. The prediction of diabetic neuropathic foot ulceration using veibration perception thresholds: a prospective study. *Diabet Care* 1994; **17**: 557–561.
3. European working group on Critical leg ischaemia. Second European Consensus Document on chronic critical leg ischaemia. *Eur J Vasc Surg* 1992; **6** (suppl. A): 15–16.
4. Walters DP, Gatling W, Mullee, Mullee MA, Hiu RD. The distribution and severity of diabetic foot disease: a community study with a comparison to a non-diabetic group. *Diabet Med* 1992; **9**: 354–358.
5. Rosen RC, Davids MS, Bohanske LM. Haemorrhage into plaster callus and diabetes mellitus. *Cutis* 1985; **35**: 339–341.
6. Martin MM. Diabetic Neuropathy. *Brain* 1953; **76**: 594–624.
7. Edmonds ME, Archer AG, Watkins PJ. Ephedrine: a new treatment for diabetic neuropathic oedema. *Lancet* 1983; **1**: 54–55.
8. Sidaway AN, Curry KM. Non invasive evaluation of the lower extremity arterial system. In: Frykberg RG (ed.), *The High Risk Foot in Diabetes Mellitus*. Edinburgh: Churchill Livingstone, 1991; 241–254.
9. Tappin JW, Pollard J, Bechett EA. Method of measuring shear forces on the sole of the foot. *Clin Phys Physiol Meas* 1980; **1**: 83–85.
10. National Institute of Clinical Excellence report. *Type 2 diabetes prevention and management of foot problems*. January 2004.
11. Cavanagh PR, Ubrecht JS. Clinical plantar pressure measurements in diabetes: rationale and methodology. In Boulton AJM, Connor H, Cavanagh PR (eds), *The Foot in Diabetes*. Blackwell: Oxford, 1994.
12. Veves A, Murray HJ, Young MJ, Boulton AJM. The risk of foot ulceration in diabetic patients with high foot pressure: a prospective study. *Diabetologia* 1992; **35**: 660–663.
13. Strandness DE Jr, Priest RE, Gibbons GE. Combined clinical and pathological study of diabetic and non diabetic peripheral arterial disease. *Diabetes* 1964; **13**: 366–372.
14. Ferrier RM. Radiologically demonstrable arterial calcification in diabetes mellitus. *Aust Ann Med* 1967; **13**: 222–226.
15. Warren S, Le Compte PM, Legg MA. *The Pathology of Diabetes Mellitus*. Philadelphia, PA: Lea and Febiger, 1966.
16. Chantelau E, Ma XY, Herrnberger S, Dohmen C, Trappe P, Baba T. Effect of medial arterial calcification on O_2 supply to exercising diabetic feet. *Diabetes* 1990; **39**: 513–516.
17. Wheelock FC, Gibbons GW, Marble A. Surgery in diabetes. In: Marble A, Krall LP, Bradley RF, Christlieb AR, Soeldner JS (eds), *Joslin's Diabetes Mellitus*. Philadelphia, PA: Lea and Febiger, 1985; 712–731.
18. Parving HH, Rasmussen SM. Transcapillary escape rate of albumin and plasma volume in short and long term juvenile diabetes. *Scand J Clin Lab Invest* 1973; **32**: 81–87.

19. Tovey FI. Establishing a diabetic shoe service. *Pract Diabet* 1985; **2**: 5–8.
20. Krupski WC, Reilly LM, Perez S, Moss KM, Crombleholme PA, Rapp JH. A prospective randomised trial of autologous platelet derived wound healin factors for the treatment of chronic non-healing wounds. *Vasc Surg* 1991; **14**: 526–536.
21. Edmonds M, Foster AVM. Diabetic foot. In: Shaw KM (eds). *Diabetic Complications*. Chichester: John Wiley and Sons, 1996; 149–178.
22. Edmonds ME, Blundell MP, Morris HE, Thomas EM. Improved survival of the diabetic foot: impact of a foot clinic. *Q J Med* 1986; **232**: 763–771.
23. Cheshire NJW, Wolfe JHN, Noone MA. The economics of femorocrural reconstruction for critical leg ischaemia with and without autologous vein. *J Vasc Surg* 1992; **15**: 167–175.
24. Cheshire NJW, Wolfe JHN. Critical leg ischaemia: amputation and reconstruction. *Br Med J* 1992; **304**: 312–315.
25. Tannenbaum G, Pomposelli GB, Maraccio EJ. Safety of vein bypass grafting to the dorsal pedal artery in diabetic patients with foot infection. *J Vasc Surg* 1992; **15**: 982–990.
26. Woelfle KD, Lange G, Mayer H, Bruijnen H, Lopreint H. Distal vein graft reconstruction for isolated tibio-peroneal occlusive disease in diabetics with critical foot ischaemia. How does it work? *Eur J Vasc Surg* 1993; **7**: 409–413.
27. Logarfo FW, Coffman JD. Vacular and microvascular disease of the foot in diabetes. *New Engl J Med* 1984; **311**: 1615–1619.
28. Gill GV, Hyatt H, Majid S. Diagnostic delays in diabetic Charcot arthropathy. *Pract Diabet Int* 2004; **21**(7): 261–262.
29. Jude EB, Selby POL, Burgess J *et al*. Biphosphonates in the treatment of Charcot neuroarthropathy: a double-blind randomised controlled trial. *Diabetologica* 2001; **44**: 2032–2037.
30. Boulton AJM. *Diabetic Neuropathy*, vol. 80 Marius Press, 1999; 155.
31. Rogers LC, Alam U, Tesfaye S, Malik RA. Treatment of painful diabetic neuropathy; a review of the most efficacious pharmacological treatments. *Practical Diabetes International* 2002; **21**: 301.
32. Oyibo SO Prasad YD, Jackson NJ, Boulton AJM. The relationship between blood glucose excursions and painful peripheral diabetic neuropathy: a pilot study. *Diabetic Medicine* 2002; **19**: 870–873.
33. Asbury AK, Fields HL. Pain due to peripheral nerve damage: an hypothesis. *Neurology* 1984; **34**(12): 1587–1590.
34. Bennett M. The LANNSS Pain Scale: the Leeds assessment of neuropathic symptoms and signs. *Pain* 2001; **92**: 147–151.
35. Tesfaye S. Diabetic neuropathy; achieving best practice. *Br. J. Diabet Vasc Dis* 2003.
36. Holland E, Bradbury R, Meeking D. Using a team approach to set up a diabetic foot referral pathway. *The Diabetic Foot* 2002; **3**: 106–110.
37. Quattrini C Tesfaye S. Understanding the impact of painful diabetic neuropathy. *Diabet Metab Res Rev* 2003; **19**: S2–S8.
38. Dyck PJ, Thomas PK. *Diabetic Neuropathy*, 2nd edn. Philadelphia, PA: WB Saunders, 1999; 262–267.
39. Benbow SJ, Daousi C, MacFarlane A. Diagnosing and managing chronic painful diabetic neuropathy. *Diabet Foot* 2004; **7**: 34–46.
40. Jarvis B Cukell AJ. Mexilitine: a review of it's therapeutic use in painful diabetic neuropathy. *Drugs* 1998; **56**: 691–707.
41. Peeler L in Dalerno E, Willens JS. *Pain Management Handbook – an Interdisciplincary Approach*, Chapter 7. Mosby: St Louis, MO; 201–229.
42. Weintraub MI, Wolfe GI, Barohn RA, Cole SP, Parry G, Hayat G, Cohen J, Page J, Bromberg MB, Schwartz SL. Static magnetic field therapy for symptomatic diabetic neuropathy; a double blind placebo-controlled trial. *Arch Phys Med Rehab* 2003; **84**(5).

43. Gonzalez J Vileikyte L, Rubin R, Leventhal. Predicators of depression in neuropathy: a longitudinal study of subjects at high risk of developing neuropathic foot ulceration. *Malvern Foot Conference*, Martin, Worcs, 12–14 May 2004.
44. Boulton AJM. Understanding painful symptomatic diabetic neuropathy. *Pract Diabet Int* 2004; **21**(4): 157–161.
45. Holland E, Land D, McIntosh S, Meeking D. Development of diabetic foot service since the introduction of a multidisciplinary diabetic foot referral pathway. *Pract Diabet Int* 2002; **19**(5): 137–138.
46. Walker S. A nurse led acupuncture service for painful diabetic neuropathy:2. *J Diabet Nurs* 2001; **5**(2): 59–62.
47. *Neuropathy; Diabetic Neuropathy – New Concepts and Insights*. Amsterdam: Elsevier; 1995; 405–408.

4

Diabetes and Autonomic Neuropathy

Andrew Macleod and **Angela Cook**

4.1   Introduction

The diagnosis of diabetic autonomic neuropathy remains in the province of the astute and experienced clinician. It is also a 'diagnosis of exclusion'; in other words it can only be made after other conditions, which may mimic the symptoms (e.g. gastrointestinal malignancy) or which may affect the autonomic nervous system (e.g. Shy Drager syndrome) have been excluded by clinical investigations (Figure 4.1).

There is no specific test that confirms the diagnosis. Autonomic function tests may be a useful aid, but must be taken in context. Tests may be 'abnormal' due to age in an elderly subject with type 2 diabetes, and a patient with type 1 diabetes may have abnormal tests but still harbour a treatable carcinoma of the caecum that is in fact responsible for the symptom of diarrhoea.

Diabetic autonomic neuropathy, however, remains a distressing condition that is often not easy to treat, and may have serious consequences for an affected individual in terms of both the quality and longevity of their life.

4.2   Causative Factors

The Diabetes Control and Complications Trial (DCCT) provided evidence that improved glycaemic control was associated with both the slowing of progression, and also a decrease in the *de-novo* development of abnormal autonomic nerve function in people with type 1 diabetes.[1] In so doing the trial confirmed the hypothesis that hyperglycaemia was a causative factor and gave promise that

Diabetes: Chronic Complications   Edited by Kenneth M. Shaw and Michael H. Cummings
© 2005 John Wiley & Sons, Ltd.

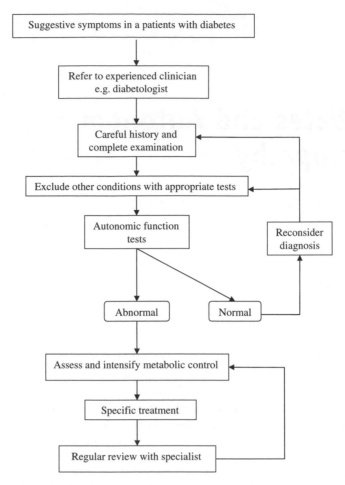

Figure 4.1   Algorithm for the diagnosis and management of diabetic autonomic neuropathy

improved blood glucose control was likely to reduce the prevalence of autonomic neuropathy, as with the other chronic complications of diabetes. Evidence also exists for type 2 diabetes.[2]

The association between hyperglycaemia and deteriorating autonomic nerve function is now universally accepted, but the mechanisms by which hyperglycaemia causes damage are still very much open to debate. Candidates include a direct metabolic insult to the nerve (whether neurones or ganglia), or to the vasa nervorum. Possible biochemical pathways include the polyol pathway, activation of protein kinase C, increased oxidative stress, with increased free radical production, and abnormalities of nitric oxide production.[3]

The typical clinical picture of diabetic autonomic neuropathy is usually seen in type 1 diabetes. Findings of an association of the clinical picture with iritis led to the hypothesis that there might be an autoimmune component to the aetiology. The beta cell is embryologically of neuroectoderm origin, and antibodies to components of the beta cell are of course well recognized in this type of diabetes. The hypothesis suggests that hyperglycaemia causes the initial damage, thus exposing intracellular components, and that an autoimmune attack against these components then accelerates the process, resulting in the clinical condition.

Antibodies directed against autonomic nerves and ganglia have been found in increased frequency in type 1 diabetes, and in increased frequency in those people with autonomic neuropathy.[4] Whether this is a causative association, or simply an unimportant by-product of autonomic nerve destruction remains to be seen.

4.3   Tests of Autonomic Function

Tests of cardiovascular autonomic function

Ewing and his colleagues in Edinburgh described a battery of five tests to assess cardiovascular autonomic nerve function in the 1970s, and some or all have since been used by many for research and clinical practice.[5] They comprise heart rate response to Valsalva manoeuvre, deep breathing and standing, and blood pressure response to standing and to hand grip. More sophisticated measures employing spectral analysis of variability of heart rate during normal breathing have also been used.

Two simple clinical tests that can be carried out in any hospital are the blood pressure and heart rate response to standing (mainly sympathetic), and the expired-to-inspired (E:I) ratio (mainly vagal).

Response to standing

In normal individuals the blood pressure is rapidly corrected on standing by baroreflex-mediated peripheral vasoconstriction and tachycardia. There may be a slight rise in blood pressure, or at the most a fall of 10 mmHg systolic pressure. The standing pressure should be measured at least 30 s after standing. Postural drops often vary considerably through the day and from week to week. An agreed definition of orthostatic hypotension is a fall on standing of systolic blood pressure of ≥ 20 mmHg, or diastolic blood pressure of ≥ 10 mmHg, accompanied by symptoms.

Expired-to-inspired heart rate ratio

The E:I ratio measures heart rate (RR interval; interval between the ECG 'R' wave of one complex and the next) from an ECG tracing during controlled deep breathing. The subject is instructed to take a deep breath lasting approximately 5 s in, 5 s out whilst resting on a couch. The shortest RR interval during inspiration (I) and the longest during expiration (E) are measured and the E:I ratio calculated. As with all tests of autonomic function, there is a decline with age: age-related normal ranges have been published.[6]

The validity of the tests is affected by the metabolic status (e.g. degree of dehydration, hyperglycaemia), time of day, time since meal and insulin, coffee intake and smoking status, and the patient's collaboration.

Other tests

Other tests of autonomic function abound in the literature, from tests that assess pupillary function to those that assess the peripheral autonomic nerves[7] (Table 4.1). Few are of use, however, in the routine clinical situation.

Table 4.1   Tests of autonomic function

	Parasympathetic	Sympathetic
Cardiovascular		
Heart rate variability	[	
Blood pressure response to standing		[
Expired-to-inspired heart rate ratio	[	
Valsalva response	[	
Pupillary		
Dark-adapted pupil diameter		[
Light reflex	[	
Gastric		
Scintigraphic or ultrasonographic test meal	[	
Peripheral		
Galvanic skin response		[(cholinergic)
Axon reflex		[

4.4   Prevalence

Widely varying estimates of the prevalence of diabetic autonomic neuropathy have been published in the literature. Calculation of the prevalence of autonomic neuropathy obviously depends on the definition of the condition, the tests used and the population studied. A European study found 16.8 per cent of patients with type 1 diabetes and 22.1 per cent patients with type 2 diabetes to have abnormalities in three out of six standard cardiovascular autonomic function tests involving heart rate variation.[8] In a community-based study in the UK (mostly type 2 diabetes), the prevalence of abnormal heart rate variability tests was 16.7 per cent.[9] A French study of diabetic patients attending seven diabetes departments (likely to have an increased prevalence of complications compared with a population-derived sample) revealed abnormal heart rate variability in 50 per cent, and even higher in those with type 1 diabetes.[10] The EURODIAB study (randomly selected type 1 diabetic patients from 31 centres in 16 European countries) examined changes in heart rate variation and blood pressure from lying to standing. An abnormality in at least one of the tests was seen in 36 per cent of patients; the heart rate variation was abnormal in 24 per cent and postural hypotension was seen in 18 per cent. Significant symptoms were seen in 18 per cent for dizziness on standing, 5 per cent for problems with bladder control, and 4 per cent for nocturnal diarrhoea.[11]

4.5　Screening for Autonomic Neuropathy

There is currently no specific treatment that might ameliorate diabetic autonomic neuropathy, other than intensifying blood glucose control, which is a goal of treatment in most people with diabetes. There is therefore currently no logic in screening asymptomatic patients for autonomic dysfunction.

The exception of course would be to screen for patients with asymptomatic coronary insufficiency (see below). There are no reports so far of clinical programmes being set up for this purpose. The standard exercise stress test may overdiagnose those with hypertension,[12] and underdiagnose high risk type 2 diabetic patients,[13] and both research groups considered that alternative screening tests should be sought.

Table 4.2　Syndromes of diabetic autonomic neuropathy

Sudomotor	Diarrhoea
Abnormal sweating	Constipation
Gustatory sweating	Faecal incontinence
Dry, warm skin	*Genitourinary*
Cardiovascular	Neurogenic bladder
Resting tachycardia	Erectile dysfunction
Postural hypotension	Retrograde ejaculation
Silent myocardial ischaemia	*Metabolic*
Anaemia	Hypoglycaemia unawareness
? Sudden death	Hypoglycaemia-associated autonomic failure
Gastrointestinal	
Oesophageal dysmotility	
Gastroparesis	

4.6 Clinical Syndromes

Sweating

Significant damage to the autonomic nerves results in reduced sweating, as seen in the dry feet of patients with severe peripheral neuropathy. Increased sweating can also occur in diabetes, particularly in the shorter nerves of the face and trunk, and is thought to be due to autonomic dysfunction. Increased sweating may also occur at night, but must be distinguished from nocturnal hypoglycaemia. Early changes in sudomotor function have been demonstrated in type 1 diabetes.[14]

This embarrassing symptom is not easy to treat but may be helped by anti-cholinergic agents. One widely recommended agent, poldine methyl sulfate, is currently unobtainable, but others, such as propantheline bromide, may help. Patients should be warned that such non-specific agents cause a dry mouth and can exacerbate postural hypotension if present. Use can be limited to provide confidence in public situations, etc.

Gustatory sweating

An unusual but relatively specific symptom of diabetic autonomic neuropathy is that of profuse sweating of the face brought about by eating ('gustatory sweating'). Again, anticholinergic agents may help.

Painful neuropathic symptoms

Painful neuropathic symptoms in diabetes do not usually correlate with the degree of histological nerve damage. There is some evidence, however, that peripheral autonomic (sympathetic) denervation may be present and may be an aetiologic factor.[15]

Gastroparesis

Diabetic gastroparesis is clinically important because it may be associated with gastrointestinal symptoms, alterations in glycaemic control, and changes in oral drug absorption. Abnormality of gastric emptying due to diabetic autonomic neuropathy can result in symptoms of nausea, bloating and vomiting. Diabetic control then becomes difficult, and ketosis worsens. Increased blood glucose levels and ketonaemia by themselves may adversely affect gastric emptying, and then exacerbate the condition, such that a vicious circle develops. Episodes may be precipitated by intercurrent infection.

It has been estimated that 50 per cent of patients with type 1 diabetes may have problems with gastric emptying, mostly as a direct result of raised blood glucose levels.[16] The interplay between the acute effect of hyperglycaemia and that of structural (and, currently, largely irreversible) nerve damage may explain why some individuals may have weeks or months of severe nausea and vomiting and then long periods without problems. There is no doubt that patients with severe autonomic nerve damage may be severely and chronically affected, but control of blood glucose and ketonaemia is still of paramount importance in such cases.

Management also consists of agents to increase gastric emptying (erythromycin, metoclopramide and domperidone). One group has advocated gastric surgery for severe chronic cases (which are rare).[17] Evidence-based studies are lacking.

A particular problem with gastroparesis may develop in pregnancy, possibly because of a combination of the autonomic dysfunction and the hyperemesis of pregnancy. Good metabolic control, i.e. blood glucose and nutrition, is essential.[18]

Case study

A 43-year-old man with 13 years of type 1 diabetes was admitted to hospital as an emergency. He had had increasingly severe bouts of vomiting for over 6 weeks, sometimes prolonged, resulting in prostration for 24–36 h. Past history included a myocardial infarction 3 years previously. He was known to have background retinopathy, and had had difficulties with poor blood glucose control for years, with HBA1c estimations of 10.7–12.6 per cent for the last 3 years despite support from the diabetes team.

On admission he was vomiting, and ketotic with a random plasma glucose of 29 mmol/l, but normal blood pH and bicarbonate. He was treated with an intravenous insulin infusion, with saline/potassium infusion, converting to dextrose/saline when the glucose had lowered. He was given parenteral antiemetics. Symptoms improved, but worsened when he was converted to subcutaneous insulin. The intravenous insulin pump was therefore reinstated. A search for infection was negative. Eventually he was controlled on his previous multiple injection regime, and discharged.

He was readmitted with the same symptoms one week later, which again settled with intensive metabolic control. He was treated with metoclopramide four times a day and low-dose erythromycin. Investigations revealed a normal abdominal ultrasound, oesophagogastroduodenoscopy and duodenal biopsy, and no lesions were seen on barium meal and small bowel meal, but gastric emptying was delayed. Expired to inspired beat-to-beat heart rate variation was abnormally diminished, and vibration threshold in both great toes was abnormally increased, with absent ankle jerks, indicative of impaired autonomic and peripheral nerve function.

A diagnosis of diabetic gastroparesis was made, and he was continued on regular metoclopramide, with intensive efforts to try to improve his blood glucose control. He has had waves of nausea since, but has had no further hospital admissions.

Diabetic diarrhoea

Intermittent profuse watery diarrhoea is well recognized symptom of diabetic autonomic neuropathy. Symptoms can be particularly distressing (see case study), and are typically worse at night. Disturbance of intestinal motility has been demonstrated, and it is suggested that small bowel bacterial overgrowth may then contribute to symptoms.[19] Again diagnosis is essentially clinical, and other causes must first be excluded with standard tests including sigmoidoscopy and colonoscopy. A careful drug history must be taken, particularly including metformin.

The symptom may be particularly refractive to treatment, but first-line therapy includes a short course of antibiotics such as tetracycline (or doxycycline if there is evidence of renal impairment) or erythromycin. Conventional treatment with codeine phosphate or loperamide may sometimes help. Anecdotal reports exist of improvement with the somatostatin analogue, octreotide; there are no randomized studies and one report documents a significant rise in blood pressure that necessitated stopping the treatment. In extreme and refractory cases surgery with formation of colostomy may be considered.

Case study

A 40-year-old woman with type 1 diabetes of 15 years' duration presented with profuse watery diarrhoea after meals, occurring every 2 or 3 days. She also has a virtually continuous feeling of nausea. After the diagnosis of diabetes, she was admitted on a number of occasions with diabetic ketosis and ketoacidosis, and has found control difficult. HBA1c values have usually been above 10 per cent. She developed retinopathy 6 years after diagnosis, evidence of peripheral neuropathy at 8 years, central cataracts at 10 years and proteinuria 11 years from diagnosis.

Investigations revealed normal abdominal ultrasound, flexible sigmoidoscopy and biopsy, oesophagogastroduodenoscopy and duodenal biopsy, and colonoscopy with interval biopsies. Despite correcting iron and folate deficiency, her haemoglobin level was constantly below the lower limit of normal. She had mild renal impairment with proteinuria despite ACE inhibitors.

Treatment was started with a short course of doxycycline, loperamide and octreotide with no benefit. Low-dose erythromycin helped the nausea, but not the diarrhoea. She is now tolerating her symptoms and has improved her glycaemic control with the support of the diabetes team.

Anaemia

In the 1990s research drew attention to the association of anaemia and diabetic autonomic neuropathy in type 1 diabetes. The suggestion was made that there might be impairment of putative sympathetic nervous control of erythropoietin release from the kidney. Such a mechanism has been suggested in 'pure' non-diabetic autonomic failure.[20] Proof of a causative relationship in people with diabetes was made difficult by the fact that a significant proportion of patients with clinical evidence of diabetic autonomic neuropathy also had evidence of significant renal damage.[21]

There is increasing evidence of a real relationship, however,[22] and also reports of symptomatic improvement, for example improvement of postural symptoms,[23] following early erythropoietin replacement. A similar correlation between evidence of autonomic nerve damage and erythropoietin deficiency has been reported in patients with type 2 diabetes.[24]

Postural hypotension

The normal response to attaining the upright posture is a slight increase in systolic pressure, mediated mainly by the sympathetic nervous system. Postural or orthostatic hypotension is usually defined as a postural drop in systolic blood pressure of at least 20 mmHg, or at least 10 mmHg for the diastolic component. Postural dizziness, disorientation or loss of consciousness can be severely disabling. The symptoms are worse on rising and in the early part of the day, and are often exacerbated following a meal, presumably due to increased splanchnic blood flow. It is also possible that autonomic neuropathy adversely affects autoregulation of cerebral blood flow, and thus the postural symptoms are exacerbated.[25] In some cases, postural symptoms may remit despite little difference in the measurement of the postural drop (see the case study).

For affected individuals, a reduction in plasma noradrenaline release with the upright posture is usually the case, but for some a paradoxical increase in noradrenaline has been reported. The authors of the report suggest that this response may be an early feature of the condition, possibly via erythropoietin deficiency (see above).[26]

Treatment consists first of simple measures, such as advice about posture, and raising the head of the bed whilst sleeping. Agents to increase blood pressure, such as fludrocortisone, may be tried, with care to avoid supine hypertension and oedema. As above, there are initial reports of success with erythropoietin replacement.

Case study

A 35-year-old woman with type 1 diabetes of 10 years' duration was seen as an emergency in the diabetes clinic. She had previously had poor blood glucose control with a number of admissions due to diabetic ketoacidosis. Her latest

HBA1c was 12.4 per cent. For the last few weeks she had experienced increasingly distressing pains in the abdomen, and both upper and lower legs, that were burning, shooting and kept her awake at night. She had experienced dizziness on standing, and although the pains had been helped by amitryptyline 25 mg o.d., the dizziness had become worse.

On examination she had hypersensitivity over the painful areas, some evidence of peripheral neuropathy, and a significant postural drop in blood pressure (110/70 mmHg lying, 90/60 mmHg standing, with resting tachycardia and no change on standing). There was no beat-to-beat variation with breathing. A diagnosis of acute painful neuropathy and acute autonomic neuropathy was made. Amitriptyline was stopped.

Over the next few days the pains became excruciating and she was admitted to hospital. The clinical features were of a persistent postural drop in blood pressure, with severe postural dizziness and tachycardia. Metabolic control was rapidly improved, fluids were encouraged, the head of the bed was raised, and she was started on low-dose fludrocortisone. Postural hypotension and dizziness improved. Pains were treated with carbamazepine, with slight improvement. Imipramine was cautiously started, with better relief of pain. Constipation became a problem and was treated with appropriate laxatives.

Over the next few weeks in outpatients her pains gradually improved, and for the first time she managed to maintain good blood glucose control. Postural symptoms had improved but blood pressure still fell from 120/80 supine to 70/50 standing. Fludrocortisone had produced ankle oedema and was phased out.

Six years later she has no pain and is fully back to work. She has minimal postural symptoms but still has a postural drop in blood pressure. She has a new relationship, and after a number of years of good blood glucose control, HBA1c levels are back up again.

Silent myocardial ischaemia

It has been suggested since the 1980s that people with diabetes may not experience angina symptoms as much as people without diabetes, despite documented coronary artery insufficiency. Clearly proof is not easy, as most subjects with coronary artery disease (CAD) are selected as a result of their symptoms. If the hypothesis is true, then those who are at an increased risk of CAD, i.e. those with diabetes, may present at a more advanced stage of the condition (if at all), and such patients should be screened and managed with assessment criteria that do not depend on symptoms. The question therefore needs to be answered.

Most researchers do now believe that there is an increased prevalence of silent myocardial ischaemia in people with diabetes. There is also increasing evidence that autonomic neuropathy may be a causative factor. In a study of patients with type 2 diabetes, 81 per cent of patients with asymptomatic coronary insufficiency had evidence of autonomic neuropathy, compared with 25 per cent of those with anginal symptoms.[27] In a review of 12 studies examining the importance of autonomic neuropathy in silent myocardial ischaemia, generally measured by exercise stress testing, five studies showed a statistically significant increased frequency of silent myocardial ischaemia in individuals with, as opposed to those without, cardiovascular autonomic neuropathy.[28] The reviewers point out, however, that some authors question whether this association is causative, suggesting instead that underlying coronary disease might be a cause of both autonomic dysfunction and silent myocardial ischaemia.

Case study

A 48-year-old woman with type 2 diabetes was admitted as an emergency to hospital having woken at 5 a.m. feeling sweaty. She went to the toilet and collapsed with loss of consciousness for probably 5 min. Her husband called the ambulance. On admission she felt faint and weak. ECG showed classical changes of an inferior myocardial infarction, and cardiac enzymes were raised. She was thrombolysed and discharged on relevant medication. Exercise testing (on beta blockers) showed clear evidence of ST segment depression without any pain. Coronary angiography revealed a tight stenosis of the dominant right coronary artery, and a stent was inserted with resolution of the stenosis.

She was understandably concerned that the cardiac rehabilitation advice focussed on what to do when chest pain was experienced, which of course she had never had. An exercise test now showed no evidence of ischaemia, and she was somewhat reassured by the plan to arrange further tests on a 6 monthly basis. Such tests have remained within normal limits for 4 years.

Sudden death

Ewing, Campbell and Clarke[29] reported on the natural history of diabetic autonomic neuropathy in 1981, and drew attention to the increased mortality of affected individuals. Their diabetic patients with abnormal autonomic function tests had a 53 per cent mortality at 5 years, compared with a mortality rate of only 15 per cent among diabetic individuals with normal autonomic function tests. Half the deaths in the former group were from renal failure, but 29 per cent suffered sudden death. Patients with classical symptoms carried a particularly poor prognosis.

The Hoorn study examined mortality in a population-derived sample of 605 individuals of 50–75 years of age. During 9 years of follow up, 43 died from cardiovascular causes. Subjects with diabetes and evidence of autonomic impairment had an approximately doubled risk of mortality.[30] In a review of the literature in 2003, Maser *et al.*[31] found 15 studies that were appropriate to include in a meta-analysis, with follow up from 0.5 to 16 years. With the exception of one study, mortality rates in people with diabetes were higher for those with autonomic neuropathy than those without, achieving statistical significance in 12 studies. For those studies that used two or more measures to define autonomic neuropathy, the pooled estimate for the increased relative risk of mortality for those with autonomic neuropathy was 3.45.

Patients with diabetic autonomic neuropathy have been shown to have reduced myocardial perfusion reserve capacity,[32] and impaired vasodilator response of coronary vessels to sympathetic stimulation.[33] The exact mechanism for the increased mortality is, however, unknown. As above, renal failure is common in these severely affected individuals, which is likely to be due to the associated chronic hyperglycaemia. The increased incidence of sudden death suggests the possibility of a fatal cardiac arrhythmia. Silent myocardial ischaemia may be a factor (see above). Although QT interval (between the ECG 'Q' wave and the 'T' wave) prolongation (increased with hypoglycaemia) has been shown to be a bad prognostic indicator in type 1 diabetes,[34] there is no good evidence that this is via autonomic neuropathy.[35]

Hypoglycaemic unawareness and hypoglycaemia-associated autonomic failure

Severe hypoglycaemia is one of the worst fears of a person with diabetes who is treated with insulin. Being unable to detect hypoglycaemia is therefore a problem of major significance. The warning symptoms of sweating, palpitation and faintness are largely produced by increased autonomic stimulation, and it has been suggested that autonomic neuropathy might be a significant factor.

More recent studies have demonstrated that there exists an acute and reversible phenomenon whereby previous hypoglycaemia lowers the threshold at which counter-regulatory responses, including catecholamines and autonomic stimulation, switch on. This has been termed 'hypoglycaemia-associated autonomic failure', or HAAF.[36] This results in both worsening of the hypo as well as lack of recognition. The phenomenon can be reversed by avoidance of hypoglycaemia.[37]

Studies in diabetic patients with and without autonomic neuropathy have failed to reveal a difference with adrenaline or symptom responses to hypoglycaemia.[38] However, data from the EURODIAB study have identified autonomic neuropathy as an independent risk factor for severe hypoglycaemia in type 1 diabetes, and in another study adrenaline responses were reported to be impaired in patients with diabetic autonomic neuropathy.[39] It seems, therefore, that the most prevalent cause of hypoglycaemic unawareness is due to the reversible, functional phenomenon (HAAF), but that if structural damage from autonomic neuropathy is present, it is likely to worsen the situation.

Hypoglycaemic unawareness is serious and of major importance to the individual with diabetes. Its presence should be checked for as part of the routine management of diabetes. When it is a problem, intensive efforts should be made to abolish hypoglycaemia,[40] and, as coined by Diabetes UK, 'make 4 (i.e. 4 mmol/l) the floor'.

Impotence

Up to 50 per cent of men with diabetes may have problems with impotence and autonomic neuropathy is a major factor[41] (see Chapter 5). Phosphodiesterase inhibitors are a major advance in this field, but the greater the evidence for clinical autonomic or peripheral neuropathy, the less they are likely to provide benefit in patients.

Neurogenic bladder (diabetic cystopathy)

Damage to the autonomic nerve supply of the bladder and urethra results in impairment of bladder sensation, increased post-void residual volume, and decreased detrusor contractility, all of which can be seen in diabetes. These abnormalities may produce repeated urinary infections and chronic retention of urine. The diagnosis is aided by urodynamic studies, and an urological opinion should be sought. Treatment includes bladder neck surgery where outlet obstruction is a problem, or intermittent self-catheterization.[42]

4.7 Conclusion

The clinical syndrome of diabetic autonomic neuropathy usually occurs in patients with long-standing and often poorly controlled diabetes. A wide variety of systems can be involved, and affected individuals often have other complications of diabetes. The condition can be at the least-distressing, at the most life-threatening. The diagnosis is often difficult and depends on clinical skill and experience. The management of affected patients is time-consuming and requires the full support of the multidisciplinary team.

References

1. Anonymous. The effect of intensive diabetes therapy on measures of autonomic nervous system function in the Diabetes Control and Complications Trial (DCCT). *Diabetologia* 1998; **41**: 416–423.

2. Gaede P, Vedel P, Parving HH, Pedersen O. Intensified multifactorial intervention in patients with Type 2 diabetes mellitus and microalbuminuria: the Steno type 2 randomised study. *Lancet* 1999; **353**: 617.

3. Cameron NE, Eaton SE, Cotter MA, Tesfaye S. Vascular factors and metabolic interactions in the pathogenesis of diabetic neuropathy. *Diabetologia* 2001; **44**: 1973–1988.

4. Muhr D, Mollenhauer U, Ziegler AG, Haslbeck M, Standl E, Schnell O. Autoantiboides to sympathetic ganglia, GAD, or tyrosine phosphatase in long-term IDDM with and without ECG-based cardiac autonomic neuropathy. *Diabet Care* 1997; **20**: 1009.

5. Ewing DJ, Martyn CN, Young RJ, Clarke BF. The value of cardiovascular autonomic function tests: 10 years experience in diabetes. *Diabet Care* 1985; **8**: 491–498.

6. Smith SA. Reduced sinus arrhythmia in diabetic autonomic neuropathy: diagnostic value of an age-related normal range. *Br Med J* 1982; **285**: 1599–1601.

7. Macleod AF, Smith SA, Cowell T, Richardson PR, Sönksen PH. Non-cardiac autonomic tests in diabetes: use of the galvanic skin response. *Diabet Med* 1991; **8** (Symposium): S67–S70.

8. Ziegler D, Gries FA, Muhlen H, Rathmann W, Spuler M, Lessmann F. Prevalence and clinical correlates of cardiovascular autonomic and peripheral diabetic neuropathy in patients attending diabetes centers. The Diacan Multicenter Study Group. *Diabet Metab* 1993; **19**: 143–151.

9. Neil HA, Thompson AV, John S, Mc Carthy ST, Mann JI. Diabetic Autonomic neuropathy: the prevalence of impaired heart rate variablilty in a geographically defined population. *Diabet Med* 1989; **6**: 20–24.

10. Valensi P, Paries J, Attali JR. French Group for Research and Study of Diabetic Neuropathy. Cardiac autonomic neuropathy in diabetic patients: influence of diabetes duration, obesity, and microangiopathic complications – the French multicenter study. *Metab Clin Exp* 2003; **52**: 815–820.

11. Kempler P, Tesfaye S, Chaturvedi N, Stevens LK, Webb DJ, Eaton S, Kerenyi Z, Tamas G, Ward JD, Fuller JH. Blood pressure response to standing in the diagnosis of autonomic neuropathy: the EURODIAB IDDM Complications Study. *Arch of Physiol Biochem* 2001; **109**: 215–222.

12. Lochen ML. The Tromso study: the prevalence of exercise-induced silent myocardial ischaemia and relation to risk factors for coronary heart disease in an apparently healthy population. *Eur. Heart J* 1992; **13**: 728–731.

13. Bacci S, Villella M, Villella A, Langialonga T, Grilli M, Rauseo A, Mastroianno S, De Cosmo S, Fanelli R, Trischitta V. Screening for silent myocardial ischaemia in type 2 diabetic patients with additional atherogenic risk factors: applicability and accuracy of the exercise stress test. *Eur J Endocrinol* 2002; **147**: 649–654.

14. Hoeldtke RD, Bryner KD, Horvath GG, Phares RW, Broy LF, Hobbs GR. Redistribution of sudomotor responses is an early sign of sympathetic dysfunction in Type 1 diabetes. *Diabetes* 2001; **50**: 436.

15. Tack CJ, Van Gurp, Holmes C, Goldstein DS. Local sympathetic denervation in painful diabetic neuropathy. *Diabetes* 2002; **51**: 3545.

16. De Block, De Leeuw, Pelckmans PA, Callers D, Maday E, Van Gaal LF. Delayed gastric emptying and gastic autoimmunity in Type 1 diabetes. *Diabet Care* 2002; **25**: 912.

17. Ejskjaer NT, Bradley JL, Buxton-Thomas MS, Edmonds ME, Howard ER, Purewal T, Thomas Pk, Watkins PJ. Novel surgical treatment and gastric pathology in diabetic gastroparesis. *Diabet Med* 1999; **16**: 488–495.

18. Macleod AF, Smith SA, Sönksen PH, Lowy C. The problem of autonomic neuropathy in diabetic pregnancy. *Diabet Med* 1990; **7**: 80–82.

19. Zietz B, Lock G, Straub RH, Braun B, Scholmerich J, Palitzsch KD. Small-bowel bacterial overgrowth in diabetic subjects is associated with cardiovascular autonomic neuropathy. *Diabet Care* 2000; **23**: 1200–120.

20. Biaggioni I, Robertson D, Krantz S, Jones M, Haile V. The anemia of autonomic failure: evidence for sympathetic modulation of erythropoiesis in humans and reversal with recombinant erythropoietin. *Ann Intern Med* 1994; **121**: 181–186.

21. Winkler AS, Marsden J, Chaudhuri KR, Hambley H, Watkins PJ. Erythropoietin depletion and anaemia in diabetes mellitus. *Diabet Med* 1999; **16**: 813–819.

22. Thomas S, Rampersad M. Anaemia in diabetes. *Acta Diabetol 2004*; **41**: 13.

23. Winkler AS, Landau S, Watkins PJ. Erythropoietin treatment of postural hypotension in anemic Type 1 diabetic patients with autonomic neuropathy. *Diabet Care* 2001; **24**: 1121–1123.

24. Spallone V, Maiello MR, Kurukulasuriya N, Barini: A, Lovecchio M, Tartaglione R. Mennuni G, Menzinger G. Does autonomic neuropathy play a role in erythropoetin regulation in non-proteinuric Type 2 diabetic patients? *Diabet Med* 2004; **21**: 1174–1180.

25. Mankovsky BN, Piolot R, Mankovsky OL, Ziegler D. Impairment of cerebral autoregulation in diabetic patients with cardiovascular autonomic neuropathy and orthostatic hypotension. *Diabet Med* 2003; **20**: 119–126.

26. Jacob G, Costa F, Biaggioni I. Spectrum of autonomic cardiovascular neuropathy in diabetes. *Diabet Care* 2003; **26**: 2174–2180.

27. Beck MO, Silveiro SP, Friedman R, Clausell N, Gross JL. Asymptomatic coronary artery disease is associated with cardiac autonomic neuropathy and diabetic nephropathy in Type 2 diabetic patients. *Diabet Care* 1999; **22**: 1745–1747.

28. Vinik AI, Maser RE, Mitchell BD, Freeman R. Diabetic autonomic neuropathy. *Diabet Care* 2003; **26**: 1553–1581.

29. Ewing DJ, Campbell IW, Clarke BF. The natural history of diabetic autonomic neuropathy. *Q J Med* 1980; **193**: 95–108.

30. Gerritsen J, Dekker JM, TenVoorde BJ, Kostense BJ, Heine RJ, Bouter LM, Heethaar RM, Stehouwer CD. Impaired autonomic function is associated with increased mortality, especially in subjects with diabetes, hypertension, or a history of cardiovascular disease: the Hoorn Study. *Diabet Care* 2001; **24**: 1793.

31. Maser RE, Mitchell BD, Vinik AI, Freeman R. The association between cardiovascular autonomic neuropathy and mortality in individuals with diabetes: a meta-analysis. *Diabet Care* 2003; **26**: 1895–1899.

32. Taskiran M, Fritz-Hansen T, Rasmussen V, Larsson HB, Hilsted J. Decreased myocardial perfusion reserve in diabetic autonomic neuropathy. *Diabetes* 2002; **51**: 3306.

33. Di Carli MF, Bianco-Batlles D, Landa ME, Kazmers A, Groehn H, Muzik O, Grunberger G. Effect of autonomic neuropathy on coronary blood flow in patients with diabetes mellitus. *Circulation* 1999; **100**: 813.

34. Veglio M, Sivieri R, Chinaglia A, Scaglione L, Carallo-Perin P. QT interval prolongation and mortality in Type 1 diabetic patients: a 5-year cohort prospective study. Neuropathy Study Group of the Italian Society of Diabetes, Piemonte Affiliate. *Diabet Care* 2000; **23**: 1381.

35. Lee SP, Yeoh L, Harris ND, Davis CM, Robinson RT, Leathard A, Newman C, Macdonald IA, Heller SR. Influence of autonomic neuropathy on QTc interval lengthening during hypoglycemia in type 1 diabetes. *Diabetes* 2004; **53**: 1535.

36. Gerich JE, Mokan M, Veneman T, Korytkowski M, Mitrakou A, Hypoglycemia unawareness. *Endocr Rev* 1991; **12**(4): 356–371.

37. Cryer PE. Diverse causes of hypoglycemia-associated autonomic failure in diabetes. *New Engl J Med* 1994; **350**: 2272–2279.

38. Kendall DM, Rooney DP, Smets YF, Bolding L, Robertson RP. Pancreas transplantation restores epinephrine. *Diabetes* 1997; **46**: 249.
39. Meyer C, Grossmann R, Mitrakou A, Mahler R, Vereman T, Gerich J, Bretzel RG. Effects of autonomic neuropathy on counterregulation and awareness. *Diabet Care* 1998; **21**: 1960.
40. Cranston I, Lomas J, Maran A, Macdonald I, Amiel SA. Restoration of hypoglycaemia awareness in patients with long-duration insulin-dependent diabetes. *Lancet* 1994; **344**: 283–287.
41. Wellmer A, Sharief MK, Knowles CH, Misra VP, Kopelman P, Ralph D, Anand P. Quantitative sensory and autonomic testing in male diabetic patients with erectile dysfunction. *BJU Int* 1999; **83**: 66–70.
42. Kaplan SA, Blaivas JG. Diabetic cystopathy. *J Diabet Complic* 1988; **2**: 133–139.

5

Diabetes and Sexual Health

Michael H. Cummings

It is now recognized that diabetes can have a profound effect on sexual health. In consequence, there has been a considerable increase in research into this area with advances in our understanding of pathophysiology and management of diabetes-related sexual health problems. Predominantly, this applies to male erectile dysfunction, where the mechanisms leading to its development are now better understood. This has resulted in the development of oral phosphodiesterase type 5 inhibitors [sildenafil (Viagra) is perhaps the most well known], which have revolutionized the management of erectile dysfunction. In contrast, although it is recognized that diabetes can have a dramatic effect on sexual function in women, research (and in consequence pathophysiology and treatment options) has been limited and this area requires further evaluation.

5.1 Male Erectile Dysfunction

Definition

Erectile dysfunction (or impotence) is defined as the inability to achieve or maintain an erection satisfactory for sexual intercourse. 'Erectile dysfunction' is currently the preferred term as it encompasses the broader problems of men and provokes less emotion than 'impotence'. In patients who present with 'impotence', it is important to ascertain their perception of the problem for two reasons: firstly, the patient may use the term inappropriately (for example equating it to painful sex or infertility) and, secondly, treatment may differ depending upon whether the achievement or maintenance of an erection is the main problem.

Diabetes: Chronic Complications   Edited by Kenneth M. Shaw and Michael H. Cummings
© 2005 John Wiley & Sons, Ltd.

Prevalence

In the largest study to investigate erectile dysfunction (ED) in diabetic males, of 541 patients interviewed, the overall prevalence of the disorder was 35 per cent.[1] The frequency of ED increased with age: 5.7 per cent of diabetic males aged 20–24 years were impotent, increasing to 52.4 per cent in the group aged 55–59 years. This population was re-interviewed 5 years later.[2] In the group of patients who were originally potent, 28 per cent had subsequently become impotent. Five factors were identified as independently predictive of the subsequent development of erectile dysfunction: age, alcohol intake, initial glycaemic control, intermittent claudication and retinopathy. Only 9 per cent of those patients who were originally impotent had regained potency, indicating the progressive nature of the disorder.

In other studies of diabetic men, the prevalence of ED has been greater than the above study, ranging up to 75 per cent.[3] Thus, ED is much more common in the diabetic compared with the non-diabetic population, where the prevalence has been reported to range between 0.1 and 18.4 per cent.[4]

There are relatively few studies that have specifically examined ED in the type 1 diabetic population but broadly speaking the prevalence seems to be similar to that of type 2 diabetic men, although a vascular aetiology is more common in the former.[5]

Who to treat

Since ED is common in diabetic men and management can be time-consuming, it is important to identify those patients who are most likely to benefit from medical intervention. In one study of 50 diabetic men who completed a questionnaire declaring ED as a problem, only 18 per cent ultimately opted for active treatment. In those patients who spontaneously complained of ED, 88 per cent undertook active treatment.[6] Thus, we would not normally advocate routine screening for the presence of ED, rather intervention should be offered to those patients who seek medical advice for the problem. Most patients are grateful to discuss the problems, however, and this should be encouraged as part of holistic care of the diabetic patient. In practice, our approach is to alert the individual with diabetes that ED is a potential complication of the condition through posters, information leaflets and verbal communication. We emphasize that it is an eminently treatable complication and discuss how it may be successfully managed. As a consequence, particularly since the launch of effective oral therapy, patients are more readily raising the issue of ED with their health care professionals.

5.2 Aetiology

Table 5.1 shows the potential causes of ED in diabetic men. The factors that are most commonly linked to its development in diabetes are abnormalities of the

Table 5.1 The aetiology of erectile dysfunction (Reproduced by permission of John Wiley & Sons, Ltd.)

Cause	Examples
Vascular	Arterial insufficiency
	Venous leakage
Neurological	Autonomic neuropathy
	Spinal cord lesions
Penile tissue abnormalities	Fibrosis of penile tissue
	Abnormalities of smooth muscle relaxation or constriction
Psychological	
Endocrine	Primary or secondary hypogonadism
	Thyroid disorders
	Hyperprolactinaemia
Renal	Renal failure and dialysis
Pharmacological	Alcohol
	Drugs
Other	Peyronie's disease
	Penile/pelvic trauma
	Phimosis
	Balanitis
	Post-inflammatory penile fibrosis
	Penile tumour
	Congenital deformity of penis

neurovascular supply to the penis or functional and structural changes within the penile tissue itself. In many instances, patients have a multi-factorial basis to their ED.

Studies of diabetic men with ED have suggested that neurological abnormalities may be present in up to 80 per cent of cases.[7] The principal abnormality lies within the parasympathetic (autonomic) nervous system responsible for tumescence whilst the sympathetic and sensory nervous systems are largely unaffected.[1,8] It must be recognized, however, that this represents a microvascular complication of diabetes which is linked in part to tissue hypoxia.

Aberrant blood flow to the penis in diabetes may be present in various forms. Diffuse atherosclerosis is a common finding in diabetes, which may affect the penile vasculature as well as other circulatory beds in the heart, brain and lower limbs. This observation supports the concept of examining other organs susceptible to vascular disease in the diabetic individual with ED. Alternatively, there may be discrete narrowings in the external iliac artery that divert blood supply away from the penile circulation (so called 'pelvic steal' syndrome).[9] However most interest has focused on the inability of the penile blood vessels to dilate in response to the appropriate vasodilatory signals (known as endothelial dysfunction), which has been demonstrated in up to 95 per cent of men with ED.[10]

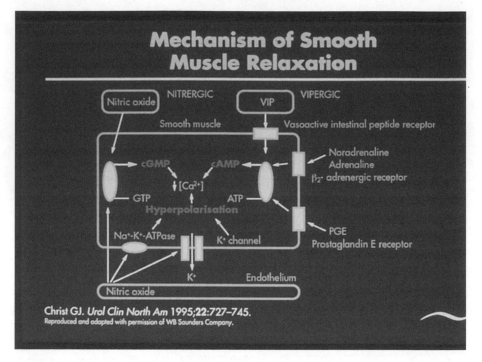

Figure 5.1 The biochemical pathways and receptors involved in penile smooth muscle relaxation (reproduced with permission from G.J. Christ, *Urol Clin N Am* 1995; **22**; 727–745)

The penile organ itself is susceptible to fibrosis within the cavernous smooth muscle, nerve fibres and blood vessels.[11] The discovery that a large number of chemical mediators are involved in the process of smooth muscle relaxation that facilitates accumulation of blood within the penis and tumescence (Figure 5.1) has led to much interest in pharmacological approaches that may correct these biochemical abnormalities. Table 5.2 highlights those mediators that have been

Table 5.2 Chemical mediators enabling smooth muscle relaxation/constriction that may be affected in diabetic men with ED (Reproduced by permission of John Wiley & Sons, Ltd.)

Relaxant	Contractile
Neuronal release	
Nitric oxide	Noradrenaline
Acetylcholine	
Vasoactive intestinal polypeptide	
Local release	
Nitric oxide	Endothelin-1
Vasodilator prostanoids	Vasoconstrictor prostanoids
Adenosine triphosphate	

Table 5.3 Drugs known to cause erectile dysfunction (Reproduced by permission of John Wiley & Sons, Ltd.)

Drug class	Examples
β-Blockers	Including eye drops; propranolol possibly the most, labetolol the least likely to cause erectile dysfunction
Diuretics	Particularly thiazides and spironolactone
Alcohol	
Antipsychotics	Phenothiazines especially thioridazine and lithium; less likely with haloperidol or pimozide
Antidepressants	Tricyclics and monoamine oxidase inhibitors
Anti-arrhythmics	Verapamil, disopyramide, flecainide, digoxin, propafenone
Lipid-lowering agents	Statins, gemfibrozil, clofibrate
Other hypotensive agents	Hydralazine, methyldopa, prazosin, clonidine
Opiate addiction	
Other	Anticonvulsants, allopurinol, anabolic steroids, baclofen, bromocriptine, cimetidine, gabapentin, ketoconazole, metoclopramide, non-steroidal anti-inflammatory drugs, oestrogens, acetazolamide

demonstrated to be abnormal in concentration or effect within the penile tissue of diabetic men with ED or rat models and form the basis of therapeutic options used in clinical management today.

Many drugs are associated with the development of ED and Table 5.3 is by no means exhaustive. In particular, drugs that treat common cardiovascular conditions or painful peripheral neuropathy and lipid-lowering drugs are common culprits in diabetic men with ED. In general, modifying or stopping a potential causative drug is only effective in restoring tumescence if there is a clear acute temporal relationship between its introduction and the development of ED.

Most studies of diabetic men with ED have shown no difference in the pituitary–gonadal axis, prolactin or thyroid abnormalities compared with potent diabetic men,[11] but the latter is more prevalent in diabetes. Balanitis is more common in diabetes in the presence of hyperglycaemia, but other conditions such as Peyronie's disease and venous leaks are present only to the same degree as in the non-diabetic population.

The majority of cases of ED in diabetes have an overt organic aetiology and this is supported by the observation that the condition rarely spontaneously improves.[1,2] It is not uncommon, however, for patients to have a concomitant secondary psychological element to their ED, for instance performance anxiety and the fear of failure. Occasionally diabetic men have a clear psychological or psychiatric condition precipitating ED which may be elicited from the consultation (see the next section).

5.3   Assessment of the Diabetic Male with ED

An accurate history, careful examination and some simple investigations should elicit the cause of erectile dysfunction and/or appropriate treatment in most diabetic patients without resorting to more complicated investigative procedures. It should be stressed that most of the assessment as to the cause of ED should be part of the regular examination of the diabetic patient. Moreover, ED should alert the health care professional to the possibility of underlying pathology elsewhere, for example, the patient may also have coronary artery disease as part of widespread vascular pathology which was not necessarily previously detected.

History

Initial useful questions

The following questions should be asked: what is the problem? Why is it a problem? What is the partner's attitude to the problem? What does the patient hope to achieve as a result of reporting the problem? These general questions will provide an overview of the problem. It may also become clear that, in some instances, the patient will not require any form of medical intervention.

Speed of onset of ED

Psychological erectile failure often presents acutely and is intermittent, whilst organic impotence has a more insidious onset and is complete.

The presence of morning, nocturnal or spontaneous erections

The ability to obtain an erection at times other than for sexual intercourse often implies a psychological origin to the problem. Nocturnal erections have been shown to be resistant to the effects of stress and are not suppressed by psychological means alone.[12]

Medical history

Since many cases of erectile failure in diabetic men are of neurological or vascular origin (or both), detailed assessment of the patient's neurovascular systems may provide clues as to the aetiology.

Neurological

The nerve supply to the bladder and the penis have the same origin (S2–4). Thus, bladder symptoms may indicate a neurological cause of ED. Evidence of autonomic neuropathy elsewhere should be sought, e.g. postural dizziness, excessive sweating, symptoms of oesophageal dysmotility or intermittent diarrhoea. Symptoms of a peripheral neuropathy, e.g. paraesthesia in a stocking distribution, may also suggest a neurological aetiology. An enquiry about the presence of symptoms arising from lesions in the cerebral cortex, e.g. cerebrovascular accident, or spinal cord, e.g. demyelination, should also be made.

Vascular

The presence of microangiopathic or macroangiopathic complications in the diabetic patient may suggest that vascular insufficiency is implicated in the cause of the patient's ED. Thus, the patient should be questioned about the presence of angina, intermittent claudication or a past history of ischaemic heart disease, peripheral vascular disease, hypertension, renal disease or retinopathy. ED in men who have two or more of the main vascular risk factors (diabetes, smoking, hyperlipidaemia and hypertension) is very likely to be due to atherosclerosis.[13]

Glycaemic control

Transient ED may occur during periods of uncontrolled diabetes and improves following improvement in glycaemic control.[14]

Endocrinology

Patients should be questioned about the presence of symptoms which may suggest thyroid disease, hyperprolactinaemia or hypogonadism.

Current health

Transient impotence may also follow an acute illness,[14] e.g. infection or myocardial infarction, and this is more often linked to a psychological origin.

Drug history

Does the introduction of any drug coincide with the time when ED was first noted? The patient should be questioned about alcohol intake since an excess of 40 units per week is a common precipitant of ED.[2]

Psychological assessment

For this purpose, it is best to interview both the patient and the partner, if they are agreeable. The assessment should focus on five main areas:[15] misconceptions about normal sexual practice, poor self-esteem and self-image, marital disharmony, and anxiety over sexual performance. A temporal relationship of a specific stress with the commencement of ED may be elicited.

Physical examination

The following systems should be carefully examined.

Genitalia

The genitalia should be inspected for congenital deformities, balanitis and phimosis. Plaques deposited along the shaft of the penis may suggest Peyronie's disease or intracorporeal fibrosis. The testes should be felt to establish normal size and consistency. Sensation over the penis may be impaired in an autonomic neuropathy. Palpation of each cavernosal artery may suggest adequate blood flow to the penis.[16] A pulsation is best felt by placing two fingers lateral to the midline, midway along the dorsum with the penis stretched away from the symphysis pubis. Neurological innervation can be tested by assessing the bulbocavernosal reflex (S2–4); pinching the glans should result in contraction of the anal sphincter. Absence of this reflex has been observed in a substantial percentage of men with primary impotence who were unable to ejaculate.[17]

Cardiovascular

Evidence of hypertension, ischaemic heart disease, peripheral vascular disease (diminished or absent peripheral pulsations, bruits, poor capillary perfusion) or cerebrovascular disease may indicate a generalized atherosclerotic process contributing to the aetiology. Postural hypotension suggests the presence of autonomic neuropathy.

Neurological

A full neurological assessment should be conducted but, in particular, the lower limbs should be assessed for the presence of a peripheral neuropathy. Impaired pain and temperature sensation may be the earliest signs of neuropathy. The presence of autonomic neuropathy can be best assessed by examining the blood pressure response to standing and sustained handgrip, the immediate heart rate response to standing, the heart rate response to the Valsalva manoeuvre and heart rate variation during deep breathing. These simple tests are described in detail elsewhere.[18] Hypothyroidism may be suspected if the reflexes are slow in relaxing.

Endocrine

Absence of secondary sexual characteristics suggests hypogonadism. Evidence of hypopituitarism should then be sought to determine if the aetiology is of a primary or secondary nature. There may be evidence of thyrotoxicosis or hypothyroidism. Hyperprolactinaemia may be suspected by the finding of gynaecomastia.

Retinal

Evidence of this microangiopathic complication may also suggest a vascular component to the aetiology of the patient's ED.

Investigations

There is no universal agreement as to the extent of investigation that should be undertaken prior to initiating treatment for ED. Our local policy has been to adopt a limited and pragmatic approach. Assessment of current and previous glycaemic control through measurement of a glycated haemoglobin or fructosamine level may help to identify those patients at risk of organic disease and be a focus of future management strategies to reduce subsequent vascular risk. However, reversal of poor chronic glycaemic control is not generally associated with improvement in erectile performance. Measurement of serum testosterone (ideally a 9 a.m. measure of free testosterone), leutinizing hormone (LH), follicle-stimulating hormone (FSH) and prolactin may identify those with a hormonal basis to their ED, although the yield in patients who appear clinically eugonad or euthyroid is relatively low. Prostatic-specific antigen (PSA) level may be measured if clinical assessment suggests underlying prostatic disease. Physical examination may lead to initiation of other investigations, particularly relevant to cardiovascular status, which may affect the appropriateness and type of treatment.

Urology departments commonly use a Doppler ultrasound technique or intracavernosal test dose of prostaglandin E1 to assess the adequacy of local penile blood flow and the likelihood of response to the latter. In the main, this applies to patients who are referred for further investigation and management if there has been a failure to respond or contra-indication to oral therapy. A large number of

Table 5.4   Investigations that may be considered to assess the aetiology of ED

Physiological tests of the autonomic nervous system (most commonly testing cardiovascular reflexes)
Detailed psychosexual assessment
Nocturnal penile rigidity studies
Cavernosography (for the possibility of veno-occlusive leakage)
Arteriography (usually only if arterial reconstruction is being considered)
MRI scan of the pituitary (if prolactinoma or secondary hypogonadism is suspected)

other investigations is available to the health care professional to further assess the nature of ED in the diabetic male (Table 5.4). It is rare that these investigations alter clinical practice, however, and their use tends to be restricted to specialist centres or for research purposes.

5.4   Discussion and Counselling

All health care professionals should at least be prepared to discuss the problem or let the patient talk about it. Simple, though perhaps obvious, questions should be a normal part of discussion and are essential for initial assessment:

- What exactly is the problem?

- Why is it a problem?

- What is your partner's attitude?

- What would you like done about it?

These questions are important in determining whether people really have erectile failure rather than some other problem such as:

- false perceptions of normality;

- pain from phimosis;

- Peyronie's disease;

- premature ejaculation.

This is important, not only in determining what the problem is, but also whether it will be necessary to refer the patient and, if so, to whom. In our experience some men may not wish to pursue physical treatment methods (as currently available), but are pleased to have had the chance to discuss the problem and have it explained and put into perspective.[6] Reassurance or advice about general health and sexual practices is appreciated and many men will come to terms with the problem. Dispelling certain myths about normal sexual practice may be helpful. Dispelling the myth that 'all men are rampant until in their coffins' may reassure a partner who may feel she is no longer desirable, or that her partner is being unfaithful. The myth that 'all women are dependent upon penetrative intercourse for satisfaction' may lead men with erectile failure to feel ashamed, not discuss their problem and completely avoid physical contact with their partner, thereby destroying a relationship unnecessarily because of performance anxiety. Sex should be for fun. It is not necessarily a performance to be judged against the often unrealistic targets seen, heard or read about in the media.

The importance of such discussions is to get the problem into perspective. It is inappropriate to refer all men to specialist surgeons or sex therapists if no real problem exists or no treatment is required. It is equally inappropriate to refer a diabetic man with organic erectile failure to a sex therapist as it is to refer a man with entirely psychological problems to a surgeon for the insertion of a prosthesis.

5.5   Management of ED in the Diabetic Male

Figure 5.2 outlines an algorithm that may be used in approaching management of diabetic men with ED. In general it is worth mentioning that improvement in chronically poor glycaemic control rarely restores potency, although ED that is associated with acute deterioration in glycaemic control may improve with resolution of the sudden metabolic deterioration. Altering or stopping causative drug treatment is a relatively uncommon therapeutic option and testosterone should be reserved for men with proven hypogonadism. The option for treating conditions such as balanitis or corrective surgical intervention is rare. Thus most diabetic men with ED need to give consideration to the therapeutic options discussed below.

Oral therapy

Phosphodiesterase type 5 inhibitors

Oral phosphodiesterase type 5 (PDE5) inhibitors are now the most commonly used oral agents in the management of ED. They enhance the availability of cyclic GMP (Figure 5.3), thereby facilitating smooth muscle relaxation and pooling of blood within the penis. Currently there are three PDE5 inhibitors available: sildenafil (Viagra),[19] tadalafil (Cialis)[20] and vardenafil (Levitra).[21] All three agents have

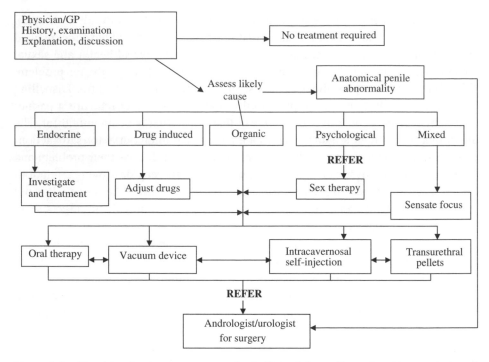

Figure 5.2 Algorithm for the management of male ED in diabetes (Reproduced by permission of John Wiley & Sons, Ltd.)

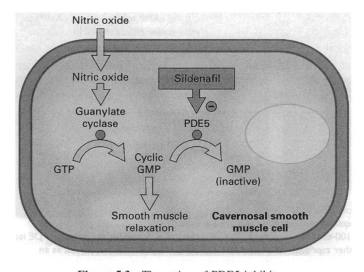

Figure 5.3 The action of PDE5 inhibitors

been shown to be effective in treating ED in diabetes and on average two out of three men respond. It is generally considered that these agents are equally as effective, although they differ in properties (e.g. sildenafil and vardenafil have a relatively short half-life of less than 4 h compared with tadalafil, with a half-life of 17.5 h) and side-effect profiles related to their ability to inhibit other PDE isoenzymes. The most common side effects shared by all three agents include headaches, flushing and indigestion, but these are usually transient and rarely inhibit long-term use. Previously concern has arisen about the potential for increasing the risk of cardiac events with the use of PDE5 inhibitors, but meta-analysis of the use of sildenafil[22] and the other PDE5 inhibitors have shown this not to be the case.

One of the most common reasons for avoiding treatment with PDE5 inhibitors is in diabetic patients who are on concomitant therapy that may potentiate a precipitous drop in blood pressure. In particular this applies to patients who are on any form of nitrate therapy or nicorandil for angina. The need for nitrate or nicorandil therapy should be reviewed in each case, but otherwise alternative treatment options should be sought.

Practical issues that need to be considered when prescribing PDE5 inhibitors include explaining the mode of action, since many men mistakenly believe oral ingestion should automatically lead to erection or improve libido. Moreover they need to be aware of 'the window of opportunity' to synchronize the most appropriate time to take their PDE5 inhibitor. The effectiveness of sildenafil and vardenafil appears to be reduced if patients have recently ingested fatty foods (which are best avoided), although this does not seem to be a concern with tadalafil. We would recommend a minimum of four attempts at achieving a desired erection when determining if the dose has been effective or whether dose titration or alternative treatments should be considered.

In state health systems such as the UK where prescriptions are rationed, patients may prefer an agent such as tadalafil with its longer duration of action and 'carry over' effect that may extend to the following day. Concerns about the increase in cost for the treatment of ED since the introduction of PDE5 inhibitors seem to be unfounded and we have demonstrated that the total costs for the treatment of ED in our district have been unchanged since their introduction.[23] Given the relatively straightforward approach to prescribing PDE5 inhibitors and the need for limited educational input compared with more invasive treatment options, initiation and monitoring of treatment is becoming more the domain of primary care health care professionals.

Apomorphine

Apomorphine (Uprima) is a sub-lingual preparation that acts as a dopamine receptor agonist within the central nervous system that facilitates the discharge of appropriate nerve signals to the penile tissue (a so-called 'central initiator').[24] There is limited available information on its effectiveness in diabetic men with ED, but it is generally regarded as less effective than PDE5 inhibitors. Again patients need to be carefully instructed on taking the medication appropriately and the potential side effects. These include nausea, vomiting, headaches and postural dizziness, but these side effects are far less common than those previously seen with much larger doses of apomorphine used to treat parkinsonism. Apomorphine may be used in patients on nitrates (classified only as a relative contraindication) with caution and appropriate assessment and monitoring. There are no rigorous studies at present that have examined the synergistic benefits of combining apomorphine treatment with PDE5 inhibitors.

Intracavernosal self-injection of vasoactive drugs

In patients who have not responded to oral therapy, this is a common second-line approach to management. When injected directly into the corpus cavernosum, the drugs produce relaxation of the smooth muscle and vasodilatation. Provided that the cavernosal tissue is responsive and that there is an adequate potential arterial blood supply, erection will ensue (Figure 5.4). Prostaglandin E1 (alprostadil) is

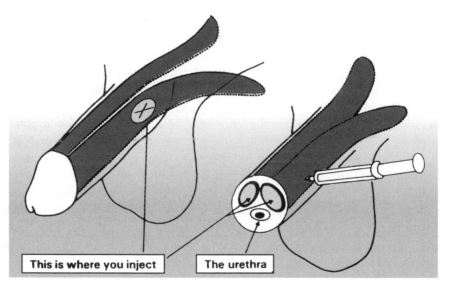

This is where you inject   The urethra

Figure 5.4 Self-administration of intracavernosal injection therapy (Reproduced by permission of John Wiley & Sons, Ltd.)

most commonly available as Caverject and is the only product actually licensed for intracavernosal self-injection within the UK. The recommended dose range is 2.5–60 µg. It is now available in a dual chamber device (powder and sterile fluid) that

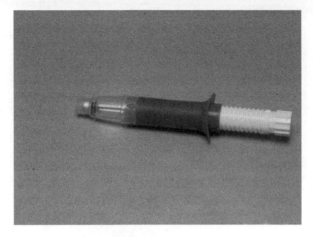

Figure 5.5 A dual chamber device for intracavernosal injection (Caverject)

can be readily mixed by twisting of the chamber cap rather than using a conventional 'syringe and needle' technique (Figure 5.5). Patients are usually taught and observed in the technique of self-injecting within the clinic setting. Evaluation of intracavernosal prostaglandin E1 suggests that this is a very effective agent for promoting tumescence in diabetic men (up to nine out of 10 may respond), with a reduced incidence of prolonged erections and of fibrosis at the injection site[25–27] compared with earlier injected agents such as papaverine. Relative disadvantages include painful erections in some men. Other side effects include prolonged erections and patients should be advised on what action to take in the event of priapism ranging from simple measures that can be undertaken at home to attending casualty for aspiration of blood from the penis, injections of an antidote (phenylephrine) or in extreme cases shunt procedures. It should be stressed that this complication is rare providing patients follow the appropriate advice over incremental dose adjustments and do not attempt multiple injections within a single 24 h period. Other recognized side effects include bruising, fibrosis and scarring, infection and syncope.

Papaverine or papaverine/phentolamine combinations may be used by some specialist centres if there is insufficient response to prostaglandin E1, although these treatments are unlicensed. Thymoxamine (Erecnos) and vasoactive intestinal polypeptide (VIP) are not available within the UK, although they are available in other European countries.

Medicated urethral system for erections (MUSE)

An alternative to self-injection is the application of pellets of prostaglandin E1 (MUSE) into the urethra (Figure 5.6). The active ingredient is absorbed in to the

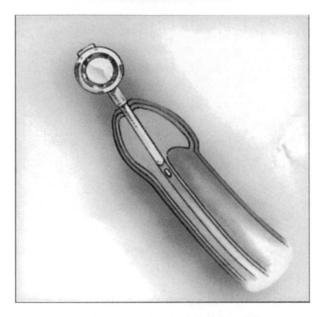

Figure 5.6   Medicated urethral system for erection (MUSE)

penile tissue, leading to smooth muscle relaxation and facilitating tumescence. As with intracavernosal therapy, time is needed to explain the technique and dose titration is required to achieve an appropriate response. We prefer to supervise patients administrating MUSE in the clinical setting to ensure appropriate application. There are no diabetes-specific studies examining the effectiveness of MUSE, although it has been shown to improve erections in a sub-group of diabetic patients within the general population.[28] Most authorities regard MUSE as less effective than intracavernosal injections and associated local pain may limit its use.

Vacuum devices

The use of vacuum tumescence devices can provide a safe and effective method of treatment for most men[29,30] and should be discussed and demonstrated as a potential first-line treatment particularly where patients wish to avoid drug therapy or where it may be contraindicated (Figure 5.7).

    The vacuum cylinder devices all work on the same principle: a vacuum tube, well lubricated, is placed over the penis with a constriction rubber band placed over the end. A battery or hand-operated pump is then attached and a vacuum produced by pumping air out. When sufficient tumescence is produced the band is slipped off on to the base of the penis, the vacuum released and the cylinder

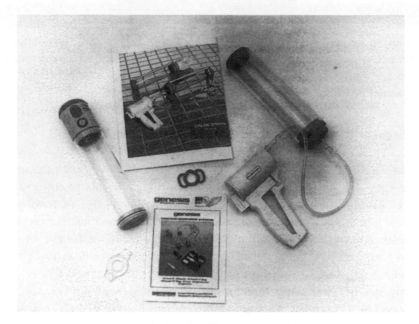

Figure 5.7   Examples of vacuum devices (Reproduced by permission of John Wiley & Sons, Ltd.)

removed. The band can safely remain in place for 30 min. They do not produce a full erection and the base will remain flaccid with the tumescent penis hanging rather than truly erect, but the result is sufficient for intercourse in 80–90 per cent of men.

Good technique is very important for success and practice may be required. Instructions should be carefully read. Most companies will provide a video instruction tape and also have a telephone helpline to guide people who are having problems. Clinicians should have available demonstration models and videos. Some patients may be put off vacuum devices because of the need for much apparatus and mess, which makes it rather obtrusive. It is important, therefore, to demonstrate the relative ease of this form of treatment. At the very least, men should be provided with company literature and order forms to give them the option of this form of treatment, as most can be ordered direct without the need for a doctor's consent or prescription. Within the UK, these devices have become available on state prescription and over a long period of time they are very cost-effective compared with drug therapy, since it is a one-off expense.

Bruising may occur with the use of a vacuum device. Significant phimosis should be excluded before recommending use as occasionally restoration of erection may produce tearing of the foreskin. Ejaculatory failure may occur due to constriction from the retention ring. Some discomfort occurs in most patients but is usually minor. Some patients find the devices rather unnatural, obtrusive and messy. They require a sympathetic and understanding partner. The 'quality' of erection is less normal than that produced by injection therapy and, although an erection may be produced in up to 100 per cent of men,[31] overall satisfaction rates may be as low as 50 per cent and, like other treatments, there is a high dropout rate over time.[29,32] Constriction rings alone may be considered in diabetic men whose predominant problem is that of maintenance of an erection.

Psychosexual therapy

In an ideal world all men should have a multidisciplinary team assessment to include specialist psychosexual advice, but unfortunately this is not possible in practice. All clinicians should therefore have some knowledge of psychological therapies, just as sex therapists will often need to advise and instruct on physical treatments. Although the majority of diabetic men with ED will have an organic basis to their problem, there will be some with primary psychological problems and most with some secondary problems. Physical treatments only restore erections but not necessarily relationships, and there will always need to be some psychological input. People with overt psychological problems or frank psychiatric disease should be referred for specialist assessment and advice before embarking upon the use of physical methods.

There are a large number of psychological therapies of varying complexity involving either the individual or the couple. From the physician's point of view, it is important to have at least a general understanding of the principles of 'sex therapy'.

Important aspects of therapies are to identify and agree a number of relevant factors:

- predisposing factors;

- precipitating factors;

- potentiating factors;

- perpetuating factors.

These should be explored, as a cue for discussion and decisions on treatment. This will be helpful in improving understanding of the problem, relieving negative thoughts of the patient and directing the physician towards the most appropriate treatments.

Sensate focusing

The physician may find it helpful to be aware, in detail, of some techniques such as the modified Masters and Johnson approach based upon 'couple therapy'.[33] This is a useful and logical treatment, not necessarily in the expectation of restoring erections but at least restoring the concept of physical enjoyment. It should encourage communication, discussion and understanding of the needs, likes and dislikes of the partners and relieve performance anxiety, an important part of the treatment programme.

The suggested programme consists of staged exercises with an agreed ban on intercourse over a set period of time. Half an hour, two or three times a week, should be devoted to these exercises, which involve three phases of sensate focusing:

- non-genital;

- genital;

- vaginal containment.

Phase 1: in the non-genital phase the couple will caress/stroke and concentrate on enjoyment of touch but not of genital areas.

Phase 2: this allows stroking and caressing to include genital areas. Intercourse should not be allowed to take place even if erection occurs in either of these stages.

The final stage: prior to allowing normal intercourse, this stage can include vaginal penetration but passively rather than with a view to orgasm or pleasing the partner. Discussion of techniques such as the modified Masters and Johnson technique should be part of any treatment discussion, even if physical methods are to be the mainstay of therapy. Such discussion helps both the physician and the patient to take a broader view of the problem and the purpose of the treatment.

Surgical treatment

Surgical treatments may be considered in three categories: correction of penile abnormalities, vascular surgery and penile prostheses.

Surgery to correct penile abnormalities

Surgery can be used to treat:

- congenital abnormalities;

- painful conditions such as a torn frenulum or phimosis;

- Peyronie's disease;

- trauma.

Clearly it is important to establish the presence of such a condition from the history, as it is most appropriate then to send the patient to a specialist surgeon/ andrologist.

Vascular surgery

This may be useful in men with congenital or traumatic vascular insufficiency and perhaps in men with major vessel disease in whom angioplasty or reconstruction may be of benefit. In general revascularization techniques remain largely experimental and positive outcomes remain disappointing. The role of venous surgery also remains much debated. Various techniques have been used to try to overcome 'veno-occlusive deficits' in men with proven good arterial inflow but inability to sustain erections due to 'venous leakage'. Long-term results from surgery have been disappointing and interest now lies in investigating the cavernosal muscle itself rather than venous channels. Men with such a problem may respond to vacuum devices or require a penile prosthesis.

Penile prostheses

The implantation of a penile prosthesis remains the mainstay of surgical treatment and with careful selection of patients is very successful in restoring the ability of an impotent man to have intercourse. It is a relatively simple operation that can be performed under general or local/regional anaesthesia.

Most surgeons would reserve the operation for men who have failed to respond satisfactorily to other forms of treatment, including oral therapy, vacuum devices or intracavernosal vasoactive drugs. This most commonly occurs in men with erectile failure from a vascular aetiology but, regardless of cause, some men will require or prefer a prosthetic implant. Careful selection and counselling is important. For efficiency this should be done before referral to specialist surgeons; Cumming and Pryor,[34] for instance, found only 16 per cent of men referred specifically for a prosthesis elected to proceed with the operation after explanation of this and alternative methods of treatment.

Prostheses are implanted as a pair and most are currently made from a silicone polymer (Figure 5.8). There are three main categories: malleable, inflatable and mechanical. Malleable prostheses are the cheapest and most reliable. The penis remains erect all the time but can be folded against the abdominal wall or thigh and is easily concealed. Mechanical and inflatable prostheses contain a mechanism, either intrinsic or attached to the device, whereby it can be kept flaccid or rigid as required. Complications include infection, mechanical failure, extrusion of the prosthesis, pain and bruising, but these are rarely serious, and significant in fewer than 5 per cent of cases with adequate precautions and an experienced surgeon.[35] High satisfaction rates are reported by both patients and their partners when carefully selected for this procedure.[36,37]

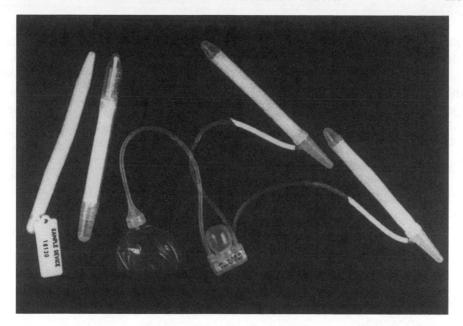

Figure 5.8 Examples of penile prostheses (Reproduced by permission of John Wiley & Sons, Ltd.)

5.6   Conclusions

The advent of PDE5 inhibitors into clinical practice has had a profound impact upon the management of ED in the diabetic male. The availability of an effective oral agent has meant that patients are not put off by the thought of invasive or obtrusive alternatives. The publicity surrounding their launch has meant that ED is far more recognized by the patient as a complication of diabetes that is amenable to successful treatment. Access to treatment has improved since most primary care organizations are able to commence treatment, although oral treatment non-responders or those in whom these agents are contraindicated will still need to have access to specialist services offering other modes of treatment. For the vast majority of diabetic men with ED, there is now effective treatment available.

5.7   Sexual Dysfunction in the Female with Diabetes

The nature of sexual dysfunction

The erectile tissue and neurological innervations of the female genitalia are homologous to the male,[38] which may contribute to the observation that diabetic women have more arousal phase dysfunction than their healthy spouses.[39] The precise prevalence of female sexual dysfunction in diabetic women remains uncertain and is quite heterogeneous in its presentation. In a recent detailed questionnaire of 270 diabetic women (and non-diabetic control subjects), it was identified that there were significant differences in perceived sexual function and attitudes towards sexual health.[40] The principal findings were that of reduced lubrication/moistness in the vaginal area, painful sex, difficulty achieving orgasm, lack of interest in sex and loss of genital sensation compared with controls. One-third of diabetic women felt that their diabetes had impacted negatively upon their choice and use of contraception and worry about fertility and fear of pregnancy led to sexual or relationship difficulties. Significantly increased problems of self-image and psychological concerns were also observed in diabetic women affecting sexual function. A further review of the limited studies of sexual dysfunction in diabetic women broadly classified the findings into four key areas.[41] The majority of studies identified a reduction in sexual desire, a decrease in vaginal lubrication and arousal, orgasmic dysfunction or anorgasmy, and dyspareunia.

Management

As health care professionals, we have traditionally focused upon identifying diabetic men with ED, but it is clear we should give every opportunity for diabetic women to express concerns about their sexual health. Whilst men typically complain about genital or ejaculatory response, females complain of inadequate enjoyment or interest and the impact upon the quality of their relationship.[42] It is

Table 5.5 Management strategies used in the treatment of female sexual dysfunction (reproduced from Meeking *et al.*[40] with permission from Blackwell Publishing Ltd.)

Type of sexual dysfunction	Potential remedy
Reduced vaginal lubrication	Water-based vaginal lubricants, local or systemic hormone replacement therapy, clitoral stimulation aids (e.g. vacuum devices), advice on the need for extended foreplay and adequate stimulation prior to sex, oral therapy, e.g. sildenafil (controversial and not proven)
Absent genital sensation	Psychosexual counselling incorporating arousal enhancement strategies and encouraging exploration of other erogenous zones, penetrative vibrating sex aids
Painful sex (dyspareunia)	Vaginal lubrication, arousal enhancement strategies (as above), consider and treat genito-urinary disease if present, reduce focus on penetrative sex
Anorgasmia	Psychosexual therapy including arousal enhancement strategies (see above), vibrating sex aids
Diminished libido	Addressing intrapersonal, interpersonal and self-image issues, treatment of concurrent sexual problems or depressive illness, hormone therapy replacement (including low-dose testosterone)

important to take an accurate history to define the problem given the hetero-geneous nature of problems that may be affecting their sex life. Inquiry should be made about causative medication and the possibility of depression. A clinical examination should routinely be conducted and the possibility of vaginal infection and/or irritation be considered.

With knowledge of the underlying problem, there are a number of approaches to treatment that may be considered (Table 5.5). There is very limited data on the use of sildenafil (Viagra) and phentolamine in the general population of women with sexual dysfunction, and findings conflict.[43–45]

References

1. McCulloch DK, Campbell IW, Wu FC, Prescott RJ, Clarke BF. The prevalence of diabetic impotence. *Diabetologia* 1980; **18**: 279–283.
2. McCulloch DK, Young RJ, Prescott RJ, Campbell IW, Clarke BF. The natural history of impotence in diabetic men. *Diabetologia* 1984; **26**: 437–440.
3. Prikhozhan VM. Impotence in diabetes mellitus. *Probl Endokrinol* 1967; **13**: 37–41.
4. Kinsey AC, Pomeroy WB, Martin CE. Age and sexual outlet. In *Sexual Behaviour in the Human Male*. Philadelphia, PA: WB Saunders, 1948; 218–262.
5. Maatman TJ, Montague DK, Martin LM. Erectile dysfunction in men with diabetes mellitus. *Urology* 1987; **29**(6): 589–592.
6. Alexander WD. The diabetes physician and an assessment and treatment programme for male erectile impotence. *Diab Med* 1990; **7**: 540–543.
7. Ellenberg M. Impotence in diabetes: the neurological factor. *Ann Intern Med* 1971; **75**: 213–219.
8. Quadri R, Veglio M, Flecchia D, Tonda L, De Lorenzo F, Chiandussi L, Fonzo D. Autonomic neuropathy and sexual impotence in diabetic patients: analysis of cardiovascular reflexes. *Andrologia* 1989; **21**: 346–352.
9. Goldwasser B, Carson CC, Braun SD, McCann RL. Impotence due to the pelvic steal syndrome; treatment by transilluminal angioplasty. *J Urol* 1985; **133**: 860–861.
10. Jevtich MJ, Edson M, Jarman WD, Herrera HH. Vascular factors in erectile failure amongst diabetics. *Urology* 1982; **19**: 163–168.
11. Cummings MH. Erectile dysfunction in diabetes. In: DeFronzo RA, Ferrannini E, Keen H, Zimmet P. *International Textbook of Diabetes*, 3rd edn. Chichester: John Wiley & Sons Ltd, 2004.
12. Karacan I, Salis PJ. Diagnosis and treatment of erectile impotence. *Psych Clin N Am* 1980; **3**: 97.
13. Virag R, Bouilly P, Frydman D. Is impotence an arterial disorder? A study of arterial risk factors in 440 impotent men. *Lancet* 1985; **I**: 181–187.
14. Podolsky S. Diagnosis and treatment of sexual dysfunction in the male diabetic. *Med Clin N Am* 1982; **66**: 1389–1396.
15. Fairbrun CG, McCulloch DK, Wu FC. The effect of diabetes on male sexual function. *Clin Endovinol Metab* 1982; **11**: 749–767.
16. Cooper AJ. Advances in the assessment of organic causes of impotence. *Br J Hosp Med* 1986; **36**: 186–192.
17. Brindley GS, Gillan P. Men and women who do not have orgasms. *Br J Psychol* 1982; **140**: 351–356.

18. Ewing DJ, Clarke BF. Diagnosis and management of diabetic autonomic neuropathy. *Br Med J* 1982; **285**: 916–918.
19. Rendell MS, Rajfer J, Wicker PA, Smith MD. Sildenafil for treatment of erectile dysfunction in men with diabetes: a randomised control trial. *JAMA* 1999; **281**: 424–426.
20. Saenz de Tejada I, Anglin G, Knight JR, Emmick J. Effects of tadalafil on erectile dysfunction in men with diabetes. *Diabetes Care* 2002; **25**(12): 2159–2164.
21. Goldstein I, Young JM, Fischer J. Vardenafil, a new highly selective PDE-5 inhibitor, improves erectile function in patients with diabetes mellitus. *Diabetes* 2001; **50**(suppl 2): 114.
22. Morales A, Gingell C, Collins M. Clinical safety of oral sildenafil citrate (Viagra) in the treatment of erectile dysfunction. *Int J Impot Res* 1998; **10**: 69–74.
23. Ashton-Key M, Sadler M, Walmsley B, Holmes S, Randall S, Cummings MH. UK department of health guidance on prescribing for impotence following the introduction of sildenafil: potential to contain costs in the average health authority district. *Pharmacoeconmics* 2002; **20**(12): 839–846.
24. Melis M, Argiolas A, Gessa G. Apomorphine induced penile erection and yawning: site of action in brain. *Brain Res* 1987; **415**: 98–105.
25. Van Ahlen H, Peskar BA, Sticht G, Hertfelder H-J. Pharmacokinetics of vaso-active substances administered into the human corpus cavernosum. *J Urol* 1994; **151**: 1227–1230.
26. Schramek P, Dorninger R, Waldhauser M, Konecny P, Porpaczy P. Prostaglandin E1 in erectile dysfunction. *Br J Urol* 1990; **65**(i): 68–71.
27. Heaton JP, Lording D, Liu SN, Litonjua AD, Guangwei L, Kim SC, Kim JJ, Zhi-Zhou S, Israr D, Niazi D, Rajatanavin R, Suyono S, Benard F, Casey R, Brock G, Belanger A. Intracavernosal alprostadil is effective for the treatment of erectile dysfunction in diabetic men. *Int J Impot Res* 2001; **13**: 317–321.
28. Padma-Nathan H, Hellstrom W, Kaiser FE. Treatment of men with erectile dysfunction with transurethral alprostadil. *New Engl J Med* 1997; **336**: 1–7.
29. Ryder RE, Close CF, Moriarty KT, Moore KT, Hardisty CA. Impotence in diabetes: aetiology, implications for treatment and preferred vacuum device. *Diabet Med* 1992; **9**(10): 893–898.
30. Vrijhof HJEJ, Delaere KPJ. Vacuum construction devices in erectile dysfunction: acceptance and effectiveness in patients with impotence of organic or mixed aetiology. *Br J Urol* 1994; **74**: 102–105.
31. Wiles PG. Successful non-invasive management of erectile impotence in diabetic men. *Br Med J* 1988; **296**: 161–162.
32. Bodansky HJ. Treatment of male erectile dysfunction using the active vacuum assist device. *Diab Med* 1994; **11**(4): 410–412.
33. Masters WH, Johnson VE. *Human Sexual Inadequacy*. London: Churchill, 1970.
34. Cumming J, Pryor JP. Treatment of organic impotence. *Br J Urol* 1991; **67**: 640–643.
35. Montague DK. Treatment of erectile dysfunction. (Editorial.) *J Urol* 1993; **150**(6): 1833.
36. McLaren RH, Barrett DM. Patient and partner satisfaction with the AMS 700 penile prosthesis. *J Urol* 1992; **147**: 62.
37. Montorsi F, Guazzoni G, Bergamaschi F, Rigatti P. Patient–partner satisfaction with semirigid penile prosthesis for Peyronies disease. A 5-year follow-up study. *J Urol* 1993; **150**(6): 1819.
38. Kolodny RC. Sexual dysfunction in diabetic females. *Diabetes* 1971; **20**: 557–559.
39. Ellenberg M. Sexual aspects of the female diabetic. *Mount Sinai J Med* 1977; **44**: 495–500.
40. Meeking DR, Fosbury JA, Cummings MH, Alexander WD, Shaw KM, Russell-Jones DL. Sexual dysfunction and sexual health concerns in women with diabetes. *Sexual Dysfunct* 1998; **I**: 83–87.

41. Enzlin P, Mathieu C, Vanderschueren D, Demyttenaere K. Diabetes mellitus and female sexuality: a review of 25 years' research. *Diabet Med* 1998; **15**: 809–815.
42. Steel JM. Diabetes and female sexuality. *Diabet Med* 1998; **15**: 807–808.
43. Basson R, McInnes R, Smith MD, Hodgson G, Spain T, Koppiker N. Efficacy and safety of sildenafil in estrogenized women with sexual dysfunction associated with female sexual arousal disorder. *Obstet Gynecol* 2000; **95**(4): S54.
44. Nurnberg HG, Hensley PL, Lauriello J, Parker LM, Keith SJ. Sildenafil for woman patients with anti-depressant induced sexual dysfunction. *Psychiatr Serv* 1999; **50**(8): 1076–1078.
45. Rosen RC, Phillips NA, Gendrano NC III, Ferguson DM. Oral phentolamine and female sexual arousal disorder: a pilot study. *J Sex Marital Ther* 1999; **25**(2): 137–144.

6

Diabetes and the Heart

Miles Fisher and **K.M. Shaw**

6.1   Introduction

Diabetes exerts its greatest adverse impact throughout the vascular system. This effect includes the well-described consequence of small vessel disease, leading to specific microvascular complications including retinopathy, nephropathy and neuropathy, but also a predisposition to premature and accelerated disorder of large blood vessels, macrovascular disease. The consequences of macrovascular disease contribute not only to significant reductions in the quality of life of the person with diabetes, but also to the most likely cause of death, and three-quarters of people with diabetes will die from cardiovascular causes. This is particularly so as advances in the management of microvascular disease now offer the real prospect that mortality and morbidity from the specific complications of diabetes can be substantially reduced. For instance, a major cause of premature mortality in type 1 diabetes over the years was diabetic nephropathy and end-stage renal failure, but there is now clear evidence that the relentless progression to renal failure can be contained and prevented by the early use of angiotensin-converting enzyme (ACE) inhibitors and the aggressive treatment of hypertension (see Chapter 2). While advanced complications from microangiopathy are potentially preventable, the ravages of large vessel disease, particularly affecting coronary, cerebral and peripheral circulation, contribute to a much greater and disproportionate effect on overall health and longevity in people both with diabetes. The careful use of multi-risk factor reduction can delay these consequences.

Diabetes: Chronic Complications   Edited by Kenneth M. Shaw and Michael H. Cummings
© 2005 John Wiley & Sons, Ltd.

6.2   Nature of the Problem

Susceptibility to coronary heart disease is increased substantially in people with both type 1 and type 2 diabetes. The development of all forms of large vessel disease is accelerated with type 1 diabetes, and is often present at diagnosis in people with type 2 diabetes. It is now well established that type 2 diabetes is part of the metabolic or insulin resistance syndrome, which comprises hypertension, dyslipidaemia, central adiposity, insulin resistance, diabetes or impaired glucose tolerance and cardiovascular disease.[1] It is less certain whether this is a simple clustering of these factors in susceptible individuals, or whether this is a single key determinant, e.g. central adiposity, or inflammation that leads to all of the other features.

The effects of diabetes on the large vessels are seen predominantly at three major sites of the cardiovascular system, namely the coronary, cerebral and peripheral arteries. Such is the process that all three sites of the circulation are often affected, conferring a triple susceptibility to arterial disease. Although the first clinical manifestation is often a specific event such as myocardial infarction, transient ischaemic attack or foot ulceration, almost certainly the initial clinical manifestation reveals the overall presence of generalized and diffuse arterial problems. Stroke is a cause of much morbidity in people with diabetes, but the cause of death in a diabetic patient who has sustained a stroke is usually related to coronary heart disease. Similarly, patients with severe leg ischaemia frequently suffer a fatal coronary event while waiting for an amputation or in the early postoperative period.

Quite often symptoms of ischaemia from differing parts of the circulation are present together, and can pose management considerations when treatments are being planned. For instance, the person with claudication of the legs as a consequence of peripheral arterial disease often gives a simultaneous history of exertional angina, only limited by the restricted mobility. If revascularization is to be considered, the problem is posed as to which should be tackled first, for relief of one then carries the prospect of aggravation of the other. The management of one particular type of large vessel disorder therefore has to take into account the effect on other aspects, which can make treatment strategies very complicated. Furthermore, even medical therapies that may be of benefit for one disorder may disadvantage another. A classical example would be the use of β-blockers for angina and hypertension, which can aggravate cold peripheries and claudication of the legs. Other than β-blockers, however, the secondary preventative strategies described later apply equally to all forms of cardiovascular disease.

Undoubtedly, large vessel disease in diabetes is becoming an increasing management problem, not only in patients with type 2 diabetes where the consequences have been only too evident, but also in patients with type 1 diabetes as the consequences of microangiopathy become more effectively controlled. Although large vessel disease is not specific to diabetes, it is greatly increased in the presence of diabetes and lesser degrees of glucose intolerance. The widespread occurrence of arterial disease within the non-diabetic population permits parallel observations to be made on the nature of the disturbance and the mechanisms contributing to its development. It is interesting that the most serious expression of large vessel disease with diabetes occurs most commonly where there is a high background instance of cardiovascular disease in the population, which allows consideration of epidemiological factors to be made. Differences in population risk would seem to be predominantly geographical, providing potential clues as to why risk varies. Susceptibility to large vessel disease is determined by a complex interaction of various factors including hereditary predisposition, disturbance of metabolic state and exposure to risk factors within the environment. For instance, the prevalence of coronary heart disease in rural India is known to be relatively small, and that reduced risk is shared by those with diabetes living in India. However, second generation people from India with diabetes living in urban UK develop severe coronary heart disease, which is presumed to be due to significant change in lifestyle or environment.

Nature of macrovascular disease

The predominant large vessel disturbance of diabetes is that of atherosclerosis or atheroma.[2] There has been considerable debate concerning whether there are specific features to diabetes, or whether it is simply an exaggeration of that seen with the non-diabetic population. Overall there is probably no major qualitative difference in the type of atherosclerosis between diabetic and non-diabetic subjects; it is predominantly an increase in the amount, extent and distribution. With diabetes, atherosclerosis is observed to be more extensive throughout the circulation with more distal involvement of blood vessels. In general, no specific arterial lesion is seen in people with diabetes, but there is evidence of more fatty streaks, intimal plaques and calcification of vessels. Plaques appear to be more prone to rupture than in non-diabetic subjects. The process of atherosclerosis is probably similar to that observed in non-diabetes, with smooth muscle cell proliferation, intimal thickening, excess collagen production and medial calcification leading to reduced blood flow.

Having recognized that the essential atherosclerotic process probably follows a similar pattern to that in non-diabetic subjects, some explanation for the increased susceptibility with diabetes must be evident. The possibility of a separate diabetic macroangiopathy, independent of but occurring in association with accelerated atherosclerosis, has been suggested, but it seems likely that some aspect of the disturbed metabolism in diabetes triggers and sustains the sequence leading to atherosclerotic change. Changes in platelet activity with increased adhesiveness and tendency to aggregation have been observed, although it is not always easy to distinguish between primary alterations as a consequence of diabetes from those changes known to occur secondarily in the presence of occlusive arterial disease. It is possible that diabetes leads to some alteration or disturbance of the endothelial barrier, thus exposing sub-intimal tissue to platelet adhesion, which in turn stimulates smooth muscle cell activity and increased uptake of low-density lipoprotein cholesterol (LDL cholesterol). As described later, the typical dyslipidaemia of diabetes includes increased amounts of small dense LDL cholesterol that are more likely to cross into the vessel wall and be retained. A recent development has been the recognition that atheroma has several strong associations with systemic inflammation, as measured by circulation concentrations of C reactive protein (CRP).[3] People who have higher levels of CRP within the normal range have a higher incidence of coronary heart disease and a higher incidence of type 2 diabetes. The interactions between CRP and other components of the metabolic syndrome are complex, and the exact role of CRP in causing atheroma, as distinct from being a marker of an ongoing atheromatous process, has yet to be defined.

Epidemiology

Often epidemiological studies do not clearly distinguish type 1 from type 2 diabetes, and so it is not entirely certain to what extent there are real differences in predisposition between these two main types of diabetes.[4] To some extent type 1 diabetes is better defined, characterized by genetic predisposition and autoimmune disturbance, while type 2 diabetes appears to be a more heterogeneous disorder including, to variable extent, the more complex metabolic syndrome characterized by the constellation of multiple cardiovascular risk factors including central obesity, hypertension, impaired glucose tolerance or diabetes and dyslipidaemia. Because of the association of this syndrome with serious risk of large vessel disease, these features have sometimes been described together as 'the deadly quartet'.

Variations in susceptibility to macrovascular disease with diabetes may have a genetic basis, result from differing metabolic disturbance of the diabetes, of which the level of glycaemic control has long been a fundamental consideration, and have many other associated risk factors, be they indicators of risk or truly causal. Some of these risk factors may in turn be directly dependent on disturbance of the diabetic state such as glycosylation and alterations of blood constituents including platelet adhesiveness. Other factors may be part of the metabolic syndrome such as hypertension, dyslipidaemia and obesity, while still others may be truly avoidable factors such as cigarette smoking, poor diet or a lack of physical activity. The differing geographical susceptibility has already been mentioned and, in general, expression of large vessel problems, particularly coronary heart disease, does correlate with the degree of atherosclerotic disease within the population concerned. However, varying prevalence between different communities living within the same regional area can also be identified, although differing genetic suscept-ibility cannot necessarily be presumed as there may be real differences in lifestyle such as diet or physical activity.

Some distinction between type 1 and type 2 diabetes seems evident from the degree of disturbed glycaemic control that correlates with the development of vascular problems. Microangiopathy seems to be primarily related to the degree of hyperglycaemia and its duration, with an uncertain genetic factor. This may well be similar in both type 1 and type 2 diabetes. For macroangiopathy the situation is less clear. By its very nature type 1 diabetes predominantly presents at a younger age than type 2, so there is opportunity for pre-clinical development of vascular disturbance. It is unusual to see serious arterial problems with teenage diabetes, or with diabetes of a few years' duration. However, serious problems, including premature coronary heart disease, may present even as young as the mid-twenties, and is detected increasingly during the third and fourth decades. With both types of diabetes a distinct threshold of hyperglycaemia predisposing to microangiopathy around 11 mmol/l is apparent, while the threshold for large vessel disease is considerably lower. Indeed, there is now evidence that the risk of development of cardiovascular disease increases within the normal, non-diabetic range. In that regard, blood glucose can be viewed in the same way as blood pressure and serum cholesterol as a continuous variable that increases cardiovascular risk rather than there being a cut-off point at which risk suddenly rises.

With type 2 diabetes large vessel susceptibility is undoubted and substantial. Often the disease process is evident at the time the diabetes is diagnosed. It is well known that the development of type 2 diabetes is insidious and the process has often been developing sub-clinically for many years prior to diagnosis. During these years, while 'the clock is ticking', vascular disease may become established, accelerated and advanced. The fact that the actual disturbance of blood sugar levels itself may not be that severe during these years argues against a direct consequence of poor glycaemic control, and suggests the involvement of an associated mechanism such as insulin resistance or inflammation. As already mentioned, type 2 diabetes may cluster with other features of the metabolic syndrome. Often the glycaemic disturbance seems relatively slight, and yet even sugars in the category of impaired glucose tolerance may be associated with severe large vessel disease.

Epidemiological studies of considerable interest have arisen from observation that nutrition during the early stages of life, particularly *in utero* and during the first year of infancy, may predispose to ill-health in adulthood. In particular low birth weight and reduced infant growth during the first year of life correlate with future development of impaired glucose tolerance, type 2 diabetes, hypertension and susceptibility to coronary heart disease. It has been postulated that under-nutrition in early life predisposes to, indeed programmes, increased prevalence of both type 2 diabetes and coronary heart disease in adults. The precise means whereby such observations may be explained are uncertain, but it does seem as though birth weight and growth during early infancy are strong indicators of future risk of developing diabetes and coronary heart disease.

Mechanisms and risk factors

The cause of increased atherosclerotic risk in diabetes is multifactorial. From understanding the processes involved in the development of atherosclerosis, along with epidemiological observations, a number of factors associated with susceptibility to premature cardiovascular disease have been identified. There is debate as to whether these factors are simply coincidental correlations or whether they truly contribute to the pathogenesis of arterial disease. As already discussed, no greater uncertainty exists than that observed with glycaemic control. With type 1 diabetes some evidence exists that the degree of cardiovascular disorder is proportional to the preceding severity of hyperglycaemia, but certainly with type 2 diabetes severe arterial disease may be associated with relatively moderate degrees of glucose intolerance.

An important aspect concerning arterial risk in diabetes relates to observed alteration in gender susceptibility. Although both males and females with diabetes carry increased risk of arterial disease, the susceptibility is particularly increased for the female patient, whose normal pre-menopausal advantage and protection from coronary heart disease is apparently lost in the presence of diabetes. Once more the explanation may be complex with interaction between obesity issues and hormonal changes. Unfavourable fat distribution, particularly central adiposity, sometimes described as android obesity, can be linked with increased androgenecity of underlying hormonal levels. In particular sex hormone binding globulin (SHBG) is inversely related to overall and upper body adiposity, and in turn associates with an atherogenic pattern of cardiovascular risk factors, including free testosterone levels, increased triglycerides and reduced HDL cholesterol.

Much of the increased prevalence of arterial disease with diabetes can be strongly related to the presence of conventional cardiovascular risk factors. Each factor confers its own increased risk, but equally the more factors that are interactive, the greater the risk becomes. The cumulative effect of multiple risk factors on the cardiovascular system is well known for the non-diabetic population, and it would seem as though the presence of diabetes at least doubles the risk for each combination of factors, be it single or multiple. Risk factors themselves simply indicate increased likelihood of cardiovascular disease, and are not necessarily causal. If risk factors are simply a reflection of increased susceptibility, it could be argued that risk factor intervention would have minimal benefit. However, the argument that risk factors actively contribute to the process of premature arterial disease is substantial, and evidence that improved outcome results from modifying and eliminating adverse risk factors is also substantial. The present understanding is that risk factors should be actively identified and individually addressed on the premiss that they are significant and potentially reversible contributors to increased cardiovascular morbidity and mortality.

6.3　Primary Prevention of Heart Disease in Diabetes

Glycaemic control

Evidence that the intensive control of hyperglycaemia reduces diabetes complications comes from the Diabetes Control and Complications Trial (DCCT) and the United Kingdom Prospective Diabetes Study (UKPDS). The DCCT reported on the effect of intensive treatment of diabetes on the development and progression of long-term complications in type 1 diabetes.[5] The 1441 patients with type 1 diabetes were studied over a mean period of 6.5 years. They were divided into two groups, a primary prevention cohort without pre-existing complications and a secondary prevention cohort of those with early complications, particularly early retinopathy. Each group was randomly assigned to either a conventionally treated group or to a more intensive therapeutic regimen. The effect on microvascular complications was striking, with substantial reduction in the development of retinopathy, nephropathy and neuropathy (see Chapter 1). However, the effect of intensive therapy on macrovascular disease was less clear. A reduction in all major cardiovascular and peripheral vascular events was observed but this did not reach statistical significance. Patients participating in the study were of relatively young age (under 39 years), which might well have influenced the outcome. There was no evidence of increased macrovascular disease with intensive insulin therapy, refuting the suggestion that injected insulin itself might predispose to increased atherosclerosis and cardiovascular morbidity.

In the UKPDS a total of 4209 patients with newly diagnosed type 2 diabetes were studied over a 10 year period.[6] Patients with a history of myocardial infarction in the last year, current angina or heart failure were excluded. A complex study design was followed, and there were multiple subgroups and sub-studies. The principle comparison was between 1138 patients who were randomly assigned to conventional treatment, and 2729 patients who were assigned to an intensive therapeutic regimen based on sulfonylurea or insulin therapy. Again, the effect of microvascular disease was striking, with substantial reductions in retinopathy and in particular the need for laser photocoagulation (see Chapter 1). Again, the effect on macrovascular disease was less clear. There was a 16 per cent reduction in myocardial infarctions in the intensive treatment group compared with the conventional treatment group, but this did not quite reach statistical significance. These patients have been followed for a few years since the end of the UKPDS, and the reduction in myocardial infarctions is now statistically significant.

In the UKPDS a major subgroup was overweight patients, defined as people who weighed more than 120 per cent of ideal body weight.[7] These patients were randomly allocated to intensive therapy with metformin in addition to randomization to either sulfonylureas or insulin. In all, 342 overweight patients were allocated to metformin, 542 to sulfonylurea therapy, 409 to insulin and 411 to the conventional treatment group. Similar reductions were seen in microvascular complications comparing metformin, sulfonylureas and insulin. An unexpected and statistically significant 39 per cent reduction in myocardial infarctions was observed in patients treated with metformin. As myocardial infarction is a common cause of death in diabetes, this translated into significant reductions in total mortality. It is because of this result that metformin is the drug of first choice for treating hyperglycaemia in overweight patients who are not controlled on diet therapy alone. The reduction in HbA1c with metformin was similar to that with sulfonylureas and insulin, so better glycaemic control was not an explanation for the finding. One possible explanation is that metformin reduces insulin resistance in the liver. The new insulin-sensitizing drugs are more potent in reducing insulin resistance, and have been shown to have beneficial effects on several components of the metabolic syndrome.[8] Studies will be completed in the next few years to see if they also significantly reduce myocardial infarctions and other cardiovascular events in people with diabetes.

Hypertension

The combination of hypertension (Table 6.1) and diabetes is a serious situation, posing increased predisposition to cardiovascular morbidity and mortality. The relationship between hypertension and diabetes has been extensively studied and there is now no doubt that, using modern definitions, hypertension does occur more commonly with diabetes, its presence does confer greater prospect of complications developing, and it must be taken as seriously as glycaemic control when planning appropriate treatment strategies for cardiovascular risk reduction. In a few rare cases the combination of hypertension and diabetes will draw attention to other underlying endocrine disorders such as acromegaly or Cushing's

Table 6.1   Pathway 1 – hypertension in diabetes

Initial blood pressure systolic >140 mmHg or diastolic >90 mmHg
Treat
Step 1: younger (e.g. <55 years) or microalbuminuria – ACE inhibitor or angiotensin receptor blocker
Step 1: older (e.g. >55 years) – diuretic
Step 2: add either diuretic or ACE inhibitor/angiotensin receptor blocker
Step 3: add calcium channel blocker
Step 4: add α-blocker or β-blocker or other agent

Target is blood pressure at least below 140 mmHg systolic and 80 mmHg diastolic. Recent guidelines suggest a treatment target of <130/80 mmHg for patients with diabetes.

disorder. Routine screening for these disorders is not normally performed in a diabetic patients with hypertension, and usually the clinical features provide sufficient suspicion of diagnosis to lead to appropriate investigation.

In the early years of type 1 diabetes blood pressure levels may not be detectably abnormal, but from late adolescence onwards a degree of elevation may be observed, and when associated with microalbuminuria, a complex interaction can ensue. Blood pressure inevitably rises with more advanced nephropathy, but even in the absence of detectable renal abnormality, high blood pressure does become more evident with longer duration of type 1 diabetes. Up to 20 per cent of type 1 patients with diabetes duration in excess of 15 years may have untreated diastolic blood pressure levels above 100 mmHg compared with 11.5 per cent of an age-matched population. With type 2 diabetes, the incidence is even greater. In the UKPDS 40 per cent of males and 53 per cent of females recorded blood pressure levels in excess of 160/95. Using the modern definition of hypertension as a blood pressure over 140/90, then three-quarters of patients with type 2 diabetes are hypertensive, and this is even higher in type 2 patients with microalbuminuria.[9]

The cause of raised blood pressure in type 2 diabetes is equally complex but almost certainly includes an essential genetic component and variable interaction with disturbance of the metabolic state, including altered endothelial function, sodium retention and possibly a consequence of hyperinsulinaemia in the insulin-resistant state. Considerable attention has been paid to the potential causative role of hyperinsulinaemia leading to hypertension, but the conclusion is still uncertain.

Whatever the mechanisms of hypertension, the effect on mortality and morbidity is beyond dispute. The presence of hypertension in diabetes is associated with reduced survival, the predominant cause of death being myocardial infarction in 40 per cent of cases. Long-term longitudinal studies show a substantial increase in mortality in the presence of both hypertension and diabetes. Furthermore, the individual increased risk of both hypertension and diabetes is not just simply doubled when the two occur together, but the combination increases the risk exponentially with greatest risk for young adults, especially women. The effect of hypertension on the development of microvascular complications is also established in that hypertension will accelerate decline in established nephropathy, eventually contributing to end-stage renal failure, as well as eye disorders such as exudative retinopathy and retinal vein thrombosis.

Treatment of hypertension in patients with diabetes can now be based on a large body of clinical evidence. This includes many studies in diabetic patients alone, such as the Hypertension in Diabetes Study (HDS), which was part of the UKPDS,[10] and careful examination of diabetic subgroups in other large studies, such as the Hypertension Optimal Treatment (HOT) study.[11] Initial management of the hypertensive diabetic patient should include advice on lifestyle, the patient being encouraged to reduce excessive weight, to modify diet by reducing sodium and saturated fat intake and to limit alcohol consumption. Pharmacological treatment is usually required, and individual patients may require multiple hypotensive agents to reach targets. Targets for the treatment of hypertension are lower than for non-diabetic subjects, and are likely to fall even further in the next few years, leading to the requirement for even more hypotensive agents.

Most groups of drugs have been shown to be of proven benefit in people with diabetes, including ACE inhibitors, angiotensin receptor blockers, β-blockers, calcium channel blockers and diuretics. The α-blocker doxazocin should not be used as first-line treatment, but may be required in combination if the patients cannot tolerate other drugs because of side-effects. A combination of ACE inhibitor or angiotensin receptor (ARA) with a thiazide diuretic is suggested as a well-tolerated starting point, especially for patients with microalbuminuria or left ventricular dysfunction. Indeed, two large studies have shown that ramipril and perindopril will reduce recurrent vascular events when given as secondary prevention in diabetic patients with existing cardiovascular disease, even if they do not have hypertension or left ventricular dysfunction.[12,13]

Dyslipidaemia

It is not always recognized that disorder of lipid metabolism is as much part of the process of diabetes mellitus as is abnormality of carbohydrate metabolism (Table 6.2). All patients with diabetes have the potential to develop abnormal lipid profiles, and at any one time as many as 25 per cent of patients attending a diabetes

Table 6.2 Pathway 2 – dyslipidaemia in diabetes

Diabetic patients with established cardiovascular disease or aged 40 years and over
Random test for total cholesterol and triglycerides
Treat all patients with simvastatin 40 mg regardless of baseline cholesterol (atorvastatin 10 mg is an alternative for primary prevention)
Repeat non-fasting total cholesterol at 1–3 months
Target total cholesterol <5.0 mol/l and 25% reduction
If target reached – repeat on an annual basis
If target not reached – increase dose *or* change to a more potent statin *or* add ezetimibe

clinic will demonstrate a lipid abnormality. In many of these the abnormality is related to poor control of diabetes, i.e. a likely secondary consequence, but in many others the level of diabetic control may be good, suggesting that hyperlipidaemia may be an independent contributory risk factor.

Although patterns may differ between type 1 and type 2 diabetes, a common basis for disturbed lipid metabolism can still be identified. Insulin deficiency is still an essential component, be it absolute (type 1 diabetes) or relative (insulin resistance/type 2 diabetes). The consequence of insulin deficiency or that of insulin resistance is much the same. Hypertriglyceridaemia predominates as insulin deficit leads to reduced lipoprotein lipase activity, and thereby decreased clearance of circulating triglycerides and low high-density lipoprotein (HDL) levels. Furthermore, increased lipolysis occurs in adipose tissue and an increase in free fatty acids is delivered to the liver, with resultant fatty change. Total cholesterol levels in people with diabetes are likely to reflect the pattern in the population at large with a contributory cardiovascular risk according to the precise level. However, with diabetes it is important to be aware that for a given level of total cholesterol the atherogenic small, dense LDL sub-fraction may be a much higher percentage than in non-diabetic subjects.

Although a variety of drugs is available for lowering abnormal lipid levels, the use of statins is preferred based on the results of many large, multi-centre randomized trials. Like the blood pressure studies these have included careful examination of diabetic subgroups, for example in the Heart Protection Study (HPS)[14] and studies performed in diabetic patients alone, for example the Collaborative Atorvastatin Diabetes Study (CARDS).[15] These statin studies in diabetes have confirmed the benefit of cholesterol lowering with statins for patients with existing cardiovascular disease, and simvastatin, pravastatin and fluvastatin are all of proven benefit for secondary prevention. More recently HPS and CARDS have proven the benefit of cholesterol lowering in primary prevention using simvastatin and atorvastatin, respectively.

Protocols for the management of diabetes now include recommendations on the measurement and treatment of lipids, although the detail concerning the age to start treatment is uncertain. All patients with existing cardiovascular disease, be it coronary heart disease, cerebrovascular or peripheral vascular disease, should be started on a reasonable dose of a statin. Current targets are to aim for a total cholesterol of below 5.0 mmol/l, and again these targets are likely to be lowered in the future. For primary prevention, the guidelines are more variable. Some consider diabetes to be a coronary heart disease equivalent, and therefore all patients should be treated with a statin regardless of whether they have existing cardiovascular disease or not. Other guidelines recommend the calculation of risk using risk tables, and intervening if the risk of a cardiovascular event if above a certain level, for example over 20 per cent risk of a cardiovascular event in 10 years. If statins are started, the targets are the same as for secondary prevention. As a minimum, a lipid profile should be checked at annual review and treatment started in patients over the age of 40, regardless of whether they have type 1 or type 2 diabetes.

The fibrate group of drugs is pharmacologically more logical to treat the typical dyslipidaemia of diabetes, as these drugs increase HDL cholesterol and decrease triglycerides. To date, evidence of benefit with these drugs on hard cardiovascular outcomes has been lacking in diabetes, but several ongoing studies should clarify the role of fibrates in the next few years. There are several new lipid-lowering drugs, including rosuvastatin, a more powerful statin, and ezetimibe, which lowers cholesterol by inhibiting the absorption of cholesterol. Short-term studies have shown improvements in the lipid profile of diabetic patients with these agents, and similar long-term studies are required examining hard cardiovascular outcomes.

Antiplatelet therapy

Antiplatelet therapy is of proven benefit for secondary prevention of cardiovascular events in people with diabetes, and is described below. The benefit for primary prevention is less certain. A meta-analysis of trials in people with diabetes demonstrated a non-significant 6 per cent reduction in events in patients who were treated with antiplatelet therapy compared with patients who received placebo.[16] Current guidelines suggest that primary prevention patients are treated according to estimated cardiovascular risk, but again there is an argument that diabetes is a coronary heart disease equivalent and therefore all diabetic patients should be started on aspirin.

Obesity

In the past it has been thought that obesity is not necessarily associated with increased cardiovascular risk, unless additional factors such as hypertension or diabetes are present. More recently, recognition that differing distribution of body fat may be relevant has led to awareness that unfavourable fat distribution is an independent indicator of cardiovascular risk. Central adiposity, with increased underlying visceral fat, sometimes known as android obesity, is associated with increased predisposition to premature cardiovascular disease, and is included as part of the metabolic syndrome. Android distribution of fat or 'apple shape' contrasts with gynoid adiposity or 'pear shape' where fat is largely concentrated on the hips, buttocks and thighs. With gynoid obesity cardiovascular complications are relatively less common. The waist–hip circumference ratio (WHR) can, therefore, be a useful indicator of risk, with a WHR greater than 0.9 pointing to the potential for significant cardiovascular problems ahead. Calculation of the body mass index (BMI) takes into account the ratio of weight to height, and allows an index of cardiovascular risk to be determined. For instance, a desirable BMI would be between 20.0 and 25.0, but once the BMI rises above 30.0 mortality risk increases substantially, with the term 'morbid obesity' being used once the BMI is in excess of 40.

With diabetes, the relationship between body weight and obesity becomes quite complex. Insulin deficiency itself is associated with a reduction in body fat and overall weight loss, while excessive insulin administration is frequently associated with unacceptable weight gain. Central obesity in diabetes, sometimes known as 'diabesity', forms part of the spectrum of the metabolic syndrome, interacting with other cardiovascular risk factors already discussed.

The cause of obesity in diabetes, as with every risk factor so far discussed, is multifactorial. Undoubtedly there is a genetic basis, and some differing metabolisms may have a basis on differing inherited traits. Having said that, there is no doubt that lifestyle factors including diet and a lack of physical activity has an equal if not greater contribution to the development of obesity and it is these that are potentially reversible.

Treatment strategies should, therefore, be directed to improving such lifestyle factors by proper dietary advice, preferably under the guidance of a dietitian, with sensible and appropriate weight reduction as required. Along with diet, a reasonable physical actvity programme should be advised in order to maintain an adequate metabolic rate, which otherwise simply diminishes as energy consumption is reduced. Despite the best of intentions with diet and exercise, long-term results are disappointing. Initial enthusiasm and motivation may well meet with success, but so often the situation is difficult to sustain and weight is slowly regained. Successful weight loss in people with diabetes will reduce the waist–hip ratio, lower the BMI, reduce blood pressure, improve lipids and improve glycaemic control in the short term. These cardiovascular risk factors all head in the right direction. A large study from the US is testing if this lifestyle intervention translates into an improved cardiovascular outcome in overweight patients with type 2 diabetes. As the changes are relatively small compared with changes in cholesterol or blood pressure with drug treatment, the study will need to follow subjects for at least 10 years to see if there is any benefit.

Pharmacological intervention for obesity requires careful consideration. Orlistat reduces the absorbtion of fat and so induces energy loss. It can help lose weight, and will also help lower blood pressure. If weight is successfully lost in people with diabetes, glycaemic control may also improve. These effects should reduce cardiovascular risk, but the cardiovascular benefits have yet to be proven in a randomized trial. Sibutramine works in a totally different way as a central appetite suppressant. It will reduce weight and may also cause slight improvements in glycaemic control. A side effect is an increase in blood pressure, so it should not be used in patients with concomitant hypertension. A large, randomized trial is underway to see if this drug reduces cardiovascular events in overweight patients, including a large proportion with type 2 diabetes.

Cigarette smoking

Of all the risk factors, cigarette smoking should be the one that is most readily reversible but in practice is less easily achieved. Indeed, the benefits of stopping smoking in diabetes may exceed other therapeutic measures for associated hypertension and dyslipidaemia. Cigarette smoking in diabetes has been linked with increased risk of developing microangiopathic complications, such as nephropathy and retinopathy, but the greatest adverse affect is on vascular morbidity and mortality. In a large cross-sectional review of a busy diabetic clinic, one of us observed a significant reduction in the number of male smokers with diabetes compared with a control non-diabetic group due to premature death![17] Cigarette smoking in combination with diabetes significantly reduces the prospects of men reaching pensionable age. Although the situation was less clear with women with diabetes, because of the then smaller numbers who smoked, it is probable that, given the increase susceptibility to coronary heart disease of the diabetic woman, the risk may be even greater. It would seem as though cigarette smoking doubles the risk of premature mortality in type 1 diabetes and, while the risk with type 2 diabetes is more complex because of the interaction with multiple risk factors, cigarette smoking continues to be a strong and separate predictor of risk in its own right.

Coronary heart events occur more frequently and with greater severity in diabetic people who smoke. It is to be regretted how often good intentions to stop smoking are expressed when serious consequences develop. Cigarette smoking not only exerts a detrimental effect on the circulation, but also adversely influences diabetic control, partly as a consequence of the direct patho-pharmacological effects of smoking, but also from associated poor aspects of lifestyle. Ironically, people with diabetes are slightly more likely to be cigarette smokers than non-diabetic subjects, and the reasons for smoking may be similar. If an effective means could be found to discourage cigarette smoking in people with diabetes before severe vascular problems develop, the dividend could be considerable. At present the best approach appears to be a combination of nicotine replacement therapy and attendance at a smoking cessation clinic, but there is little specific data in diabetic patients.

6.4 Management of Heart Disease in Diabetes

The heart in diabetes can affected by several pathologies, in addition to coronary heart disease, including diabetic autonomic neuropathy and a diabetic cardiomyopathy. The various clinical expressions of coronary heart disease, angina, acute myocardial infarction/acute coronary syndromes and heart failure, all occur more commonly with diabetes, often presenting at an earlier age and with greater severity. Epidemiological observations indicate geographical variation in the frequency of clinical coronary heart disease, being as low as 6 per cent prevalence in Japan, in contrast to the much higher proportion in the Western world. This would suggest an environmental lifestyle effect, probably of a dietary nature, for the apparent protection is lost when Western lifestyle is adopted. The earlier presentation of coronary heart disease in type 1 diabetes is often evident by the fourth decade and not infrequently significant disease may present at an even younger age, including women well before the menopause. With type 2 diabetes some evidence of underlying coronary disorder, be it clinical or electrocardiographic, is frequently present at diagnosis, often in association with detectable cerebrovascular and peripheral arterial disease of the legs as well. All coronary manifestations occur more frequently, and to greater severity, while the trend towards a decline in the coronary mortality rate of the population at large is not as yet so clearly evident for people with diabetes.

Stable angina

The classical description of exertional constricting central chest tightness may not always be obtained in people with diabetes, despite severe underlying coronary heart disease (Table 6.3). Symptoms described may be much more subtle and atypical, including simple fatigue, which may obscure an accurate diagnosis. This

Table 6.3 Pathway 3 – angina in diabetes

New-onset chest pain or chest tightness

Refer to cardiology for exercise testing

Confirmation of diagnosis and risk stratification

If low risk – medical treatment

If high risk – coronary angiography

Aspirin, β-blocker (or rate-limiting calcium channel blocker), ACE inhibitor, control of hypertension (pathway 1), statin (pathway 2)

Worsening symptoms

Re-refer cardiology

is particularly so when the patient is young and female, and the diagnosis does not seem probable. However, unusual chest symptoms, particularly with an exertional component, must be taken seriously, for it is known that 'silent' (asymptomatic) ischaemia frequently occurs, and clinically evident angina is likely to represent the tip of the iceberg.

When angina is suspected, or as part of a review screening protocol for asymptomatic patients, a resting electrocardiograph may be helpful. ST segment or T wave abnormalities may be detected, suggesting underlying ischaemia, and not infrequently signs of previously unsuspected old myocardial infarction may be present. Patients with suspected coronary heart disease should be referred to a cardiologist for full assessment, including stress testing. This enables confirmation of the diagnosis and stratification of the severity of the disease, which will then lead to either initial medical therapy, or invasive investigation with coronary arteriography with a view to possible coronary artery surgery or percutaneous coronary intervention. Positive exercise tests may be found in up to 25 per cent of asymptomatic patients with type 2 diabetes and also in a significant proportion of patients with type 1 diabetes with duration of diabetes longer than 15 years. Such is the extent of potential silent coronary heart disease that could be identified by exercise testing, that the need for and implications of investigating for asymptomatic coronary disease are hotly debated. At the moment there is no clear evidence that those without symptoms but with positive exercise ECGs are any better managed for that knowledge, and it is doubtful whether present resources could meet the potential demand of further investigation including angiography, and its treatment consequences such as coronary artery bypass surgery.

Drug therapy for angina in diabetes is similar to that given to non-diabetic angina sufferers, but some care needs to be taken. This is particularly so with use of β-blockers, which can modify hypoglycaemic symptoms and impair recovery from hypoglycaemia in patients who are treated with insulin if non-selective β-blockers are used. The use of cardioselective β-blockers, e.g. atenolol, bisoprolol or metoprolol, is recommended. In the presence of peripheral arterial disease, claudication and cold feet can be aggravated by β-blockers. Despite this, β-blockers should not be regarded as contraindicated for people with diabetes as in addition to providing useful control of the symptoms of angina they also improve the long-term survival and reduce the risk of sudden death. Calcium channel blockers and the potassium channel blocker nicorandil have no significant deleterious effect in diabetes and may be used, while oral nitrates can be particularly helpful. Patients with worsening angina, not responding to increasing doses of anti-anginal medication, should be re-referred to a cardiologist and considered for further investigation, including repeat stress testing and coronary arteriography if necessary. It should be recognized that coronary arteriography is likely to show more severe changes involving all three main vessels and of a more diffuse and distal nature. The latter does create greater technical difficulty for successful coronary bypass grafting, but in some instances lesions may be only proximal, and thereby amenable to either angioplasty or bypass surgery. Coronary artery bypass grafting is the preferred treatment for diabetic patients who have triple vessel disease, as several studies have shown an improved survival compared with percutaneous coronary interventions.[18]

Acute coronary syndromes

Of all coronary heart disease manifestations, much has been reported concerning myocardial infarction in diabetes, emphasizing the increased susceptibility to heart attacks and increased severity of such, with greater frequency of associated problems and higher consequent mortality. As with angina, the presentation of acute myocardial infarction may be very atypical, often with reduced or absent chest pain, which in turn can lead to failure to establish the correct diagnosis, thereby delaying management and initiation of inappropriate treatment, and in particular thrombolytic therapy. Patients may present with rather vague chest symptoms, including a feeling of breathlessness rather than pain, and not uncommonly with non-specific symptoms including loss of well-being and tiredness. Deterioration in diabetic glycaemic control may have happened for no obvious explicable reason, and diabetic ketoacidosis may be precipitated by an otherwise silent underlying myocardial infarction. These considerations have important implications for the early management of acute myocardial infarction and so a high index of suspicion must be maintained with diabetes presenting acutely with non-specific symptoms or unexplained loss of control.

Increased risk of myocardial infarction with diabetes is a reflection of the accelerated and more severe atherosclerotic occlusive disease process of the coronary arteries. The complications of myocardial infarction including arrhythmia, conduction disorders, congestive cardiac failure and cardiogenic shock occur more commonly. The infarct size is not larger in people with diabetes, and there may be an adverse contribution from autonomic neuropathy and the diabetic cardiomyopathy. Mortality from acute myocardial infarction is significantly worse in diabetes, with approximately twofold increased mortality risk in men, and threefold in women. Immediate mortality from myocardial infarction in diabetes is as high as 34 per cent compared with about 18 per cent when diabetes is not present, while at 6 months up to 50 per cent mortality has been reported. This increased mortality is likely to reflect the greater severity of underlying coronary disease and the fact that more complications occur during the acute stages. However, recent studies from coronary care registries have shown that one reason for the increased mortality is a failure to use appropriate and proven therapies. Beta-blockers are often omitted because of worries about masking hypoglycaemic symptoms, but as mentioned above, these drugs improve long-term survival. The other erroneous fear is of retinal haemorrhage with thrombolytic therapy in patients with diabetic retinopathy. This is no more likely to occur in a diabetic patient than in a non-diabetic patient, and is exceedingly rare. If anything, thrombolytic therapy saves more lives in people with diabetes so it should be administered along with aspirin whenever indicated.[19]

Other therapeutic aspects in the management of myocardial infarction should follow general principles and guidelines. It is worth commenting that the use of ACE inhibitors may have a special beneficial role with diabetes. It is now routine practice to introduce an ACE inhibitor at an early stage of acute myocardial infarction, particularly full-thickness anterior and for those considered at risk of left ventricular dysfunction. By its nature, those with diabetes are more likely to be in this category, such that early usage of ACE inhibitors should have a significant impact on outcome, particularly towards lessening of cardiac failure and reduction in subsequent mortality.

Hyperglycaemia, with a blood sugar in excess of 11 mmol/l, is commonly found in patients with acute myocardial infarction presenting to coronary care units. In the past this was attributed to 'stress' hyperglycaemia. The precise nature of stress hyperglycaemia is still debated but in many instances observed hyperglycaemia can be a genuine indication of preceding, unsuspected diabetes. In others this is a manifestation of impaired glucose tolerance that is unmasked by the hormonal response to the infarction. Of all patients leaving a coronary care unit, one-third will have diabetes, one-third impaired glucose tolerance or impaired fasting glucose, and only one-third will have totally normal glucose tolerance. Whatever its nature, hyperglycaemia is associated with a more adverse outcome in proportion to the level of blood sugar. Hyperglycaemia associates with other adverse metabolic disturbances, including increased release of free fatty acids and increases in counter-regulatory hormones, which in turn may aggravate tendency to arrhythmias and impair myocardial contractility, leading to greater severity of cardiac failure.

Coronary care unit management of acute myocardial infarction complicating diabetes requires particular skilled management and locally agreed guidelines for glycaemic control should be made available. All patients should have an initial blood sugar estimation on admission to the coronary care unit. Levels above 11 mmol/l should be actively treated. In most cases, low-dose intravenous insulin infusion according to written protocols will prevent metabolic decompensation and worsening hyperglycaemia. One study from Sweden demonstrated that a high-dose insulin infusion protocol followed by intensive subcutaneous insulin for at least 3 months reduced mortality compared with patients who were given conventional treatment.[20] A larger, multinational study from the same researchers did not confirm these findings, and the exact role of intensive insulin therapy following myocardial infarction remains uncertain. In practical terms, for those where the blood sugar rapidly falls back to single figures, oral hypoglycaemic agents may be continued, while for those whose sugars remain elevated, subcutaneous insulin remains the preferred therapy of choice. During convalescence, review of treatment and a possible return to oral agents can be made.

Diabetic patients suffering acute myocardial infarction may require a longer stay in hospital before discharge home, especially if they have been started on insulin. Most patients will have echocardiography and an exercise test before discharge. Treatment on discharge should include low-dose aspirin therapy, a β-blocker, a statin and in all probability an ACE inhibitor as well. At follow-up review, other potential contributory risk factors should be addressed and duly dealt with as needed. Consideration of further cardiac investigation should follow the same criteria as for non-diabetic subjects, and the presence of diabetes should not be regarded as a specific contraindication. Each patient deserves consideration on an individual basis.

Cardiac failure

Primary myocardial failure in diabetes is a major determinant of cardiac morbidity and mortality. The risk of cardiac failure for men with type 1 diabetes increases twofold and for women fivefold, once more identifying the greater adverse effect of diabetes in the female. Similarly, with type 2 diabetes increased predisposition to angina and myocardial infarction is accompanied by greater severity of heart failure. Coronary artery disease significantly contributes to the development of heart failure either acutely with myocardial infarction or more insidiously in association with ventricular remodelling. In many cases, underlying myocardial ischaemia remains undetected, until cardiac failure presents. The diabetic myocardium may show diffuse fibrotic changes as a consequence of ischaemia, and possible preceding, subclinical microinfarcts. The aetiology of heart failure in diabetes is complex. Apart from the clear effect of coronary disease, myocardial function may be impaired directly by adverse metabolic changes, such as glycoprotein deposition, and possibly in some instances by the development of microangiopathy. As a result of such observations the term 'diabetic cardiomyopathy' has been introduced, when primary myocardial disturbance is often out of proportion to the severity of the coronary disease. Obesity, hypertension and nephropathy contribute their own aggravating influence to the already compromised myocardium, and thereby accelerate decline in cardiac function.

Acute left ventricular failure is a common consequence of acute myocardial infarction in diabetes. The degree of left ventricular dysfunction is the major determinant of outcome following myocardial infarction and is responsible for the greater case fatality observed with diabetes, both in the immediate post-myocardial infarction period and over subsequent months.

In some patients the development of heart failure is more insidious, presenting without history of angina or infarction. Slowly developing exertional breathlessness can sometimes be difficult to distinguish from angina, when central chest tightness may be felt more as difficulty in breathing than as pain as such. Exertional breathlessness, particularly on walking up an incline or upstairs and on lying flat in bed at night, should raise suspicion of underlying left ventricular failure. Signs on physical examination may be very deceptive initially, with no clinical evidence of cardiac enlargement, while added chest sounds may be minimal or even absent. Similarly, the chest X-ray may prove unhelpful, as the stiffer diabetic myocardium reduces cardiac enlargement, giving rise to apparently normal cardiac size. Electrocardiography may show the presence of previously unsuspected old myocardial infarction, but often only non-specific abnormalities are present. If heart failure is suspected, the patient should undergo echocardiography. This can be helpful in revealing a reduced left ventricular ejection fraction, the presence of wall motion abnormalities if there has been a previous myocardial infarction, and an overall global restriction of myocardial function. Echocardiography will also exclude valvular heart disease as a cause for the cardiac failure.

With the passage of time, heart failure becomes more manifest, often associated with relapsing bouts of acute left ventricular failure, leading to recurrent hospital admission with severe distressing breathlessness. With prompt intravenous diuretic therapy it is remarkable how often quick return to apparent normality can be achieved once fluid overload has been relieved. With such admissions it is unusual to find significant ECG or cardiac enzyme changes. The episode simply reflects the increasing incapacity of the diabetic myocardium to cope with maintaining a normal cardiac output and circulation. Left ventricular dysfunction predominates during the early stages of chronic failure in diabetes, but eventually congestive cardiac failure ensues with added right heart features, particularly oedema of the legs, becoming increasingly apparent.

Loop diuretics have a first line role in the management of heart failure, either intravenously for acute episodes or as maintenance therapy for the control of symptoms once the situation is stabilized. Loop diuretics improve symptoms, but do not affect the overall poor prognosis. The most significant development in the treatment of heart failure with diabetes has been the introduction of ACE inhibitor therapy, which does seem to have a special role in diabetes. Indeed, the usage of ACE inhibitor therapy has altered the natural history of heart failure, leading to longer survival and patients with chronic heart failure, interrupted by episodes of acute left ventricular failure, surviving and struggling on, whereas previously they would not have done so. Most diabetic patients with heart failure can be treated successfully with ACE inhibitor therapy, but the commencement of treatment should follow the usual precautions with the first administration, namely starting with a small test dose under supine conditions. Patients who have been treated with diuretics for some time prior to initiation of ACE inhibitor therapy should probably have the first dose administered under hospital supervision, usually as a day case. Potassium levels and urea and electrolytes should be monitored, and usually the ACE inhibitor effect is sufficient to offset the potassium-losing effect of loop diuretics. The ACE inhibitor should be discontinued if there is a significant deterioration in renal function. The main side effect of ACE inhibitor therapy is cough, and if this occurs the use of an angiotensin receptor blocker is an alternative. Indeed, recent studies suggest an extra benefit if ACE inhibitors and angiotensin receptor blockers are combined. The other drug that has transformed the management of cardiac failure is β-blockers, and carvediolol and metoprolol are of proven benefit in improving survival.

The potassium-sparing diuretics can be particularly prone to causing hyperka-laemia in diabetes and should be avoided when an ACE inhibitor is introduced. As heart failure progresses and resultant increasing doses of diuretics are used, the electrolyte balance becomes even more difficult to maintain. Fluid accumulation in extravascular tissues increases while the intravascular compartment becomes increasingly hypovolaemic. Addition of a thiazide to existing loop diuretic therapy can sometimes enhance diuresis and improve symptoms of cardiac failure, but in due course these electrolyte difficulties become increasingly difficult to manage.

Revascularization of the myocardium generally offers little benefit to the patient with cardiac failure as the coronary circulation is diffusely narrowed and so coronary bypass surgery is unlikely to be helpful in this late situation. Occasion-ally, however, a single lesion can be identified that can be amenable to percuta-neous coronary intervention or bypass grafting. Cardiac transplantation may be considered for severe end-stage diabetic heart failure, and indeed a number of diabetic patients have received heart transplants. However, the presence of diabetes poses special difficulties, and the presence of other long-term complications or infections seriously affects outcome, such that cardiac transplantation is not always regarded as a treatment option available for the diabetic patient.

6.5 Secondary Prevention of Heart Disease in Diabetes

The diabetic patient who has survived an acute coronary event or who has stable angina pectoris requires the long-term continuation of therapies that have been proven to improve the prognosis and reduce the subsequent mortality. This will include β-blockers, ACE inhibitors, statins and antiplatelet therapy. Until recently aspirin was the main form of antiplatelet therapy for the treatment of coronary disease, with the recognized side effects of dyspepsia and gastrointestinal bleeding. Clopidogrel is a new agent that inhibits platelets in a different way to aspirin. It causes slightly less gastrointestinal bleeding than aspirin, and in one large trail, including patients with diabetes, was slightly more effective than aspirin in reducing the risk of recurrent cardiac and cerebrovascular events. As it is a new drug it is more expensive than aspirin, and its use is restricted to certain groups of patients. It is also of benefit when given in addition to aspirin for the treatment of unstable angina, and following percutaneous coronary interventions.

6.6 Conclusions

Large vessel disease contributes significantly to premature morbidity and mortality in diabetes. Already known to be a substantial problem in people with type 2 diabetes, its importance with type 1 diabetes becomes increasingly apparent as microvascular complications become more effectively contained. Large vessel disease in diabetes is probably the most important clinical challenge ahead, and the outstanding complication to be addressed. The present tragedy is that so often major circulatory disorder develops during a long and silent period such that, when clinically evident, the consequences are already severe, critical and potentially life-threatening. It is a tragedy that first clinical awareness of such problems may be an extensive myocardial infarction, refractory cardiac failure or even sudden death. Can this be avoided?

To truly undertake prevention much more understanding of the mechanisms involved in the process of atherosclerosis in diabetes will need to be determined. The underlying causes and mechanisms are still far from clear. Undoubtedly there will be genetic factors, but how are they mediated? What is the relationship to disturbed metabolism and the metabolic syndrome? What is the relationship to hyperglycaemia when impaired glucose intolerance can be associated with advanced arterial risk? Does good control of blood sugar make any difference or should we be striving for as near normal blood sugar levels as possible? Can good control of diabetes be commenced as early as possible in the process? Yet the clinical presentation is often preceded by a long silent period of metabolic risk, increasing the difficulties of early intervention. Type 2 diabetes, in particular, poses a complex situation. The concept of the insulin resistance syndrome is deliberated and the effects of consequent hyperinsulinism debated.

Apart from metabolic considerations, acquired or environmental factors do seem very important. Studies relating to nutrition *in utero* and early childhood have drawn attention to a striking potential relationship to future development of arterial disease and/or diabetes, but still do not adequately explain acquisition of risk when moving from low- to high-prevalence areas. It is probable that a fundamental genetic susceptibility interacts with environmental factors, and it is with the latter that the best immediate prospect of successful preventive measures is offered.

Central obesity is a bad indicator of health and associates with risk of diabetes and vascular morbidity. Avoidance and reduction of obesity should be strongly encouraged by dietary measures and appropriate physical activity. By a careful and sensible combination of dietary adjustment and increased physical activity or exercise, weight can be lost, but sustaining the progress is difficult and often disappointing. Maintaining support and motivation is an important part of management in this respect. Cardiovascular risk factors significantly contribute to the development of arterial problems in people with diabetes, and risk factor assessment, including hypertension, dyslipidaemia and cigarette consumption, should be an important part of any guidelines being followed for the management of diabetes.

The sooner that large vessel disease is detected, the earlier effective interventional therapy can be initiated. A high degree of suspicion should be held for those at potential risk, especially those with strong family histories of diabetes and associated vascular disease. Once the presence of diabetes is known, review protocols should include essential screening guidelines for the early detection of large vessel disorder. Reduction and indeed prevention of large vessel arterial disease with diabetes still pose considerable difficulties in the present management of patients with diabetes, but, by these means of early risk factor intervention and early detection, there is reasonable optimism that dividends can be obtained and the more serious consequences lessened. It is to be hoped that the recent considerable advances in the management of microvascular disease of diabetes will find parallel observation for that of large vessel disease as well.

References

1. Reaven GM. Role of insulin resistance in human disease. *Diabetes* 1988; **37**: 1595–1607.
2. Kannel WB, McGee DL. Diabetes and cardiovascular disease. The Framingham Study. *JAMA* 1979; **241**: 2035–2038.
3. Tall AR. C-reactive protein reassessed. *New Engl J Med* 2004; **350**: 1450–1452.
4. Garcia MJ, McNamara PM, Gordon T, Kannel WB. Morbidity and mortality in diabetics in the Framingham population. Sixteen year follow-up study. *Diabetes* 1974; **23**: 105–111.

5. The Diabetes Control and Complications Trial (DCCT) Research Group. Effect of intensive diabetes management on macrovascular events and risk factors in the Diabetes Control and Complications Trial. *Am J Cardiol* 1995; **75**: 894–903.
6. UK Prospective Diabetes Study (UKPDS) Group. Intensive blood-glucose control with sulfonylureas or insulin compared with conventional treatment and risk of complications in patients with type 2 diabetes (UKPDS 33). *Lancet* 1998; **352**: 837–853.
7. UK Prospective Diabetes Study (UKPDS) Group. Effect of intensive blood-glucose control with metformin on complications in overweight patients with type 2 diabetes (UKPDS 34). *Lancet* 1998; **352**: 854–865.
8. Haffner SM, Greenberg AS, Weston WM, Chen H, Williams K, Freed MI. Effect of rosiglitazone treatment on nontraditional markers of cardiovascular disease in patients with type 2 diabetes mellitus. *Circulation* 2002; **106**: 679–684.
9. Tarnow L, Rossing P, Gall MA, Nielsen FS, Parving HH. Prevalence of arterial hypertension in diabetic patients before and after JNC-V. *Diabet Care* 1994; **17**: 1247–1251.
10. UK Prospective Diabetes Study Group. Tight blood pressure control and risk of macrovascular and microvascular complications in type 2 diabetes: UKPDS 38. *Br Med J* 1998; **317**: 703–713.
11. Hansson L, Zanchetti A, Carruthers SG *et al.* for the HOT Study Group. Effects of intensive blood-pressure lowering and low-dose aspirin in patients with hypertension: principal results of the Hypertension Optimal Treatment (HOT) randomised trial. *Lancet* 1998; **351**: 1755–1762.
12. Heart Outcomes Prevention Evaluation (HOPE) Study Investigators. Effects of ramipril on cardiovascular and microvascular outcomes in people with diabetes mellitus: results of the HOPE study and MICRO-HOPE substudy. *Lancet* 2000; **355**: 253–259.
13. The European trial on reduction of cardiac events with perindopril in stable coronary artery disease investigators. Efficacy of perindopril in reduction of cardiovascular events among patients with stable coronary artery disease. *Lancet* 2003; **362**: 782–788.
14. Collins R, Armitage J, Parish S, Sleigh P, Peto R for the Heart Protection Study Collaborative Group. MRC/BHF Heart Protection Study of cholesterol-lowering with simvastatin in 5963 people with diabetes: a randomised placebo-controlled trial. *Lancet* 2003; **361**: 2005–2016.
15. Colhoun HM, Betteridge DJ, Durrington PN, Hitman GA, Neil HAW, Livingstone SJ, Thomson MJ, Mackness MI, Charlton-Menys V, Fuller JH, on behalf of the CARDS Investigators. Primary prevention of cardiovascular disease with atrovastatin in type 2 diabetes in the Collaborative Atorvastatin Diabetes Study (CARDS): multicentre randomised placebo-controlled trial. *Lancet* 2004; **364**: 685–696.
16. Antithrombotic Trialists' Collaboration. Collaborative meta-analysis of randomised trials of antiplatelet therapy for prevention of death, myocardial infarction, and stroke in high risk patients. *Br Med J* 2002; **324**: 71–86.
17. Bulpitt CJ, Shaw KM, Hodes C, Bloom A. The symptom patterns of treated diabetic patients. *J Chron Dis* 1976; **29**: 571–583.
18. The Bypass Angioplasty Revascularization Investigation (Bari) Investigators. Comparison of coronary bypass surgery with angioplasty in patients with multivessel disease. *New Engl J Med* 1996; **335**: 217–225.
19. Fibrinolytic Therapy Trialists (FTT) Collaborative Group. Indications for fibrinolytic therapy in suspected acute myocardial infarction: collaborative overview of early mortality and major morbidity results from all randomised trials of more than 1000 patients. *Lancet* 1994; **343**: 311–322.
20. Malmberg K for the DIGAMI (Diabetes Mellitus, Insulin Glucose Infusion in Acute Myocardial Infarction) Study Group. Prospective randomised study of intensive insulin treatment on long term survival after acute myocardial infarction in patients with diabetes mellitus. *Br Med J* 1997; **314**: 1512–1515.

7

Diabetes and the Brain

Iain Cranston

7.1 Introduction

The vast array of glucose-regulatory systems in mammalian physiology gives lie to the importance of glucose as the primary energy source for the brain; indeed uninterrupted cerebral glucose delivery is a cornerstone of the survival of the genera. Diabetes (and its treatment) results in a far greater variability than normal in the glucose levels seen by the brain, and one might therefore expect to see disruptions its normal functioning. The fact that until recently this dysfunction was not a readily recognized phenomenon speaks more to the insensitivity of the tools used to monitor and measure cerebral function and the motivation to do so, rather than to the relative importance of glucose flux compared with other cognitive modifiers for cerebral function.

An individual's cerebral function is a result of a complex amalgamation of cerebral anatomy and physiology with significant modifiers of education, mood, age, sex, blood flow and many other factors including metabolic variability (Figure 7.1). Thus cerebral function varies across populations and (over time) within individuals.

Diabetes can either directly or indirectly potentially have significant impact on all the modifiers of cerebral function (lost education due to hospitalization is an example of an indirect effect), thus differentiating the direct metabolic effects of diabetes on the central nervous system (CNS) from its indirect effects can be difficult. However directly attributable effects would include those cognitive impairments induced acutely by glucose fluctuation (most notably episodic hypoglycaemia), and any potential long-term results of such fluctuation (far more difficult to measure), as well as those seen as a result of chronic hypergly-caemia and the multiple vascular risks associated with the metabolic syndrome and

Diabetes: Chronic Complications   Edited by Kenneth M. Shaw and Michael H. Cummings
© 2005 John Wiley & Sons, Ltd.

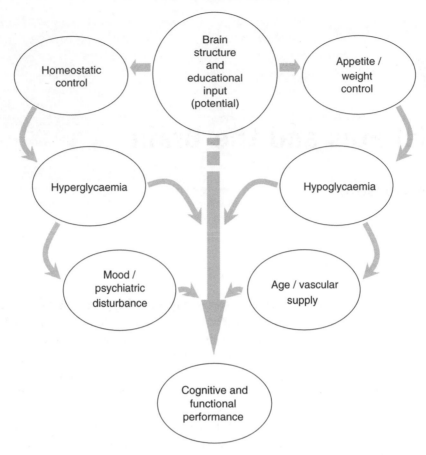

Figure 7.1　Complex interplay of some of the factors determining cerebral performance

type 2 diabetes in particular. This review will deal primarily with these areas most closely associated with our day-to-day clinical understanding of diabetes, touching additionally on other areas of association between diabetes and its potential effects on the brain and its function.

7.2　Cerebrovascular Disease and Diabetes

The acute effects of atherosclerotic cerebrovascular disease can be profound and, if survived, produce long-term defects in cerebral function with potential loss of independence, resulting in an immense personal, social and financial burden. Worldwide there are approximately 4.5 million deaths from stroke each year, making it the second most common cause of death.[1] In the Western world between 2 and 5 in 100 adults die each year from stroke, and in the UK approximately

5 per cent of the total national health budget is consumed by stroke disease (£1.6 million per 100 000 population per annum).[2] Epidemiologic studies of the prevalence of stroke reliably identify diabetes (predominantly type 2) as a risk factor for ischaemic stroke alongside others such as smoking and hypertension and, although the strength of its association is variable across studies, possibly dependant upon the degree of co-factor analysis undertaken, most suggest a risk between two and three times that for the non-diabetic population. Whilst co-factor analysis attempts to separate risk attributable to single aspects of pathogenesis, this may actually underestimate the role of diabetes in stroke disease, as so many of the recognized risk factors co-exist in the population with type 2 diabetes. Pathological examination of brain tissue from stroke victims with diabetes reveals a much higher rate of small vessel disease of the penetrating vessels supplying the thalamic and sub-thalamic areas, with increased rates of 'lacunar' infarction as a result.[3] This penetrating vessel disease appears to be a specific pathological entity resulting from hypertrophy of the medial smooth muscle, with subsequent replacement by protein and vessel occlusion, known as hyaline arteriosclerosis. The large vessel disease in diabetic patients does not seem to differ from the large vessel disease seen in non-diabetic patients. The exact frequency with which such disease affects the population as a whole is at present less clear than previously. Increased rates of high definition cerebral imaging (with MRI particularly) are highlighting that a significant level of such vascular disease can exist without the development of focal neurological signs that may give rise to a clinically identifiable ischaemic syndrome.

The data for stroke risk in type 1 diabetes is less clear, but those with long-standing disease would appear to have a total mortality risk of approximately 10 per cent as a result of stroke disease. Although the studies looking at haemorrhagic stroke are few, no such association has been described for diabetes as a risk factor for either intracranial or sub-arachnoid haemorrhage.[4]

In addition to the greater incidence of ischaemic cerebrovascular disease seen in diabetic patients, the outcome following such a cerebrovascular event is worse in patients with diabetes, with higher mortality, less complete and slower recovery and higher final dependence scores for equivalent sized infarcts occurring in the non-diabetic population.[5] The absolute glucose level during and after an ischaemic event is an important determinant of this risk, possibly by increasing lactate-associated acidity in ischaemia-affected areas secondary to increased anaerobic metabolic activity because of the hyperglycaemia. Animal models where focal ischaemia is induced artificially confirm this and show that hyperglycaemia present at the time of the insult increases the size of the resulting infarctive area. Indeed the presenting glucose level at the time of cerebral infarction has been shown to be an independent risk factor for the outcome of the event in a recent meta-analysis,[6] although such associative studies cannot easily determine if the glucose is the cause of the higher morbidity, or if the more severe the insult the higher the 'stress response' glucose level. It seems likely that both these possibilities are likely to contribute a part of the total association seen, linking presenting glucose values to outcome after stroke. Although glucose levels may be the most obvious abnormality in diabetic patients, there are other potentially important factors that also contribute to the poor outcome, such as platelet dysfunction, hyperviscosity and coagulation cascade deficits resulting in hyper-coagulability, endothelial dysfunction and decreased fibrinolytic activity.[7] In the management of vascular risk in diabetic patients all these factors should be taken into account and addressed if overall risk is to be reduced and outcome improved.

7.3 Primary Prevention of Stroke in Diabetes

In order to justify an aggressive interventional approach to the primary prevention of strokes in the diabetic population (as the epidemiology would seem to indicate the need), in an ideal world one would be able to quote data from large primary prevention studies. However one cannot at present time quote direct diabetes-related evidence in support, as many aspects of such a multi-faceted approach have been proven to be of benefit only in studies excluding diabetic subjects. It is, however, a reasonable extension of currently available data to utilize those interventions shown to be of benefit in atherosclerotic disease elsewhere (e.g. aspirin in primary prevention of ischaemic heart disease) in this population with such a high overall risk.

Recent guidelines looking into the management of vascular risk in diabetes populations[8] have all been in agreement that the risk level for non-diabetic patients receiving secondary preventative measures is equivalent to the primary risk level of patients with diabetes and any other vascular risk marker, even though these individuals may not have direct evidence of active vascular disease. Whilst this primary prevention risk case has been made most persuasively for coronary heart disease, it is also almost certainly true for cerebrovascular disease. The risk reduction strategies to prevent cerebrovascular disease will be familiar from other parts of this text; however they can be summarized in pathway management diagrams such as Figure 7.2.

One aspect of such multiple risk reduction strategies is particularly worthy of specific mention, namely the process of anticoagulation in individuals with non-valvular atrial fibrillation (nAF). Within the UKPDS cohort, individuals suffering such nAF were at an eight times greater risk of developing ischaemic stroke. In the Stroke Prevention in AF trial[9] it was shown that, if nAF is present in patients with other vascular risks [age >75, hypertension, congestive cardiac failure/left ventricular (CCF/LV) dysfunction on echo, previous thromboembolic disease], then warfarin should be commenced, targeting the INR to 2.0–3.0, as it results in a 75 per cent reduction of the stroke risk. If no other risk factors exist or if the risks of anticoagulation are considered too high, then aspirin may be a reasonable alternative risk reduction strategy, although the evidence that it actually

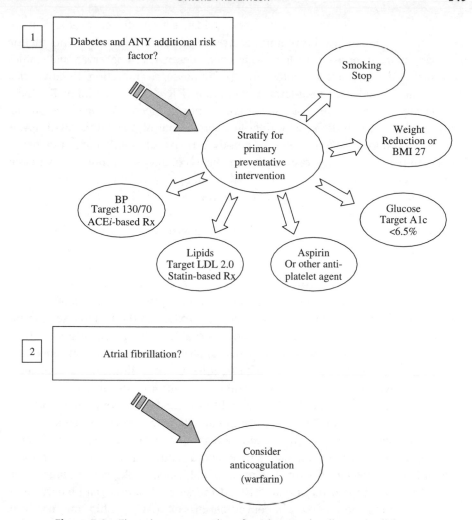

Figure 7.2 The primary prevention of cerebrovascular disease in diabetes

prevents ischaemic stroke is, surprisingly given the good coronary heart disease (CHD) data, lacking. Patients with AF and valvular disease should also be anti-coagulated (and be considered for interventional surgery for their abnormal valve).

7.4 Stroke Prevention

Whilst primary stroke prevention is a key strategy for the management of those at recognized risk, its component parts are perhaps more universally practised in those who have already experienced cerebral symptoms (previous stroke, transient ischaemic attack or amaurosis fugax), i.e. secondary stroke prevention. In this category specifically there is now far more evidence from diabetes sub-groups of large intervention studies. Preventing recurrence of stroke in a diabetic population is of particular importance, as diabetes has been described in observational studies as a major determinant of both early (<30 days) re-infarction [relative risk (RR) = 1.85][10] and later long-term re-infarction (RR = 1.7);[11] additionally, there is some suggestion that this risk can be significantly reduced from an observational study of patients with diabetes in tight glycaemic control post-stroke, with levels seen in this group close to those of the non-diabetic population.[12] Further evidence for the importance of glucose control in the secondary prevention of vascular complications comes from the UKPDS, although with the differences seen between different methods of glucose control (particularly with respect to the benefits for those overweight patients randomized to therapy with metformin), it is not at present possible to say if it is the glucose control or the method of achieving it which confers the benefit.

Lipid therapies, particularly those lowering LDL cholesterol, have had a high profile in secondary macrovascular disease prevention since 1994, and the publication of the '4S' study using simvastatin,[13] the diabetic cohort of this study[14] having over 200 patients, confirmed and extended the benefits seen in the non-diabetic population. The CARE study with 588 diabetic subjects and LIPID (with 782), both using pravastatin, reported approximately 25 per cent reductions in the total atherosclerotic disease with treatment, and following on from these data there have been other numerous studies confirming the benefits. A meta-analysis and review[15] highlighted this benefit in secondary prevention, reporting a 22 per cent risk reduction for any stroke in patients with known vasvcular disease treated with statins, 28 per cent for thromboembolic stroke, 23 per cent for non-fatal stroke and 2 per cent for fatal stroke, and a reduction of 6 per cent in those without known vascular disease. The recently published stroke data from the HPS study further confirmed this trend.[16] Blood pressure reduction [particularly with thiazide diuretics and angiotensin-converting enzyme (ACE) inhibitors] has been shown to play a major role in the secondary prevention of stroke disease, with relative risk figures of between 0.5 and 0.7 reported across most of the larger studies where diabetic sub-populations were involved. UKPDS, using either captopril or atenolol as the primary therapeutic agent, showed a relative risk of 0.56 in diabetic patients allocated to tighter hypertension control, whilst the sub-population of HOPE, using ramipril,[17] reported a relative risk of 0.67. Notably, the PROGRESS[18–20] study, using a combination of perindopril and indapamide in secondary stroke patients with no particular blood pressure entry criteria, showed a risk reduction of 28 per cent in stroke over a 4 year period (number needed to treat for 5 years to save a life = 11), with a 16 per cent reduction in dependency/ disability and a 13 per cent reduction in dementia following stroke.

Thus there is good evidence for the use of all the traditional macrovascular disease-modifying agents in diabetes for the secondary prevention of stroke and the burden of disease associated with it. Additionally, there are specific protective strategies that should be considered such as antiplatelet agents. The commonest of these in clinical practice is of course aspirin, which in the antiplatelet trialists' meta-analysis[21] was shown to carry a risk reduction of approximately 25 per cent with equal effect in diabetic and non-diabetic patients (thus an absolute benefit that is higher in diabetic patients who are at greater baseline risk). There is, however, continuing debate as to the most appropriate dose of aspirin to use in diabetic patients, with the evidence recommending anything between 50 and 325 mg daily, and the complications data suggesting that mid- to lower-range doses may confer less risk of gastrointestinal bleeding. There has been concern that 'aspirin resistance' may exist in diabetic patients, although clinical studies have yet to determine any outcome benefit of higher aspirin doses, resulting in the fact that clinical practice doses remain for the most part in the 75–150 mg per day range. There are of course other antiplatelet agents with the most well-publicised at present being clopidogrel (a thienopyridine which inhibits platelet aggregation induced by adenosine phosphate), for which evidence has been gathered from the CAPRIE study.[22] The data from this study has been widely presented as showing a 0.5 per cent additional risk reduction for patients on clopidogrel as opposed to aspirin, with complications and side-effects very similar to those with aspirin; however, interestingly the data from this study for true secondary stroke prevention ($n = 6400$) do not show any superiority of effect. It may, however, be prudent to use this therapy in particularly at-risk groups, for example where there has been a recurrent event despite aspirin in an individual who is not suitable for anticoagulation.[23] Ticlodipine (another member of the same class) has also been trialled with some success in stroke disease, although its side-effect profile has significantly limited its usefulness in routine clinical practice. A more traditional antiplatelet agent that has been in clinical use for many years is dipyridamole, which used in monotherapy is probably less effective than aspirin (although remains a useful alternative in those who are unable to take aspirin, with a lower gastrointestinal side-effect rate than clopidogrel, but with potential side effects of headache); however, its recent evidence base would suggest that, when used in combination with low-dose aspirin, it has a significant additive effect, almost doubling the risk reduction seen with aspirin 50 mg alone.[24] Following on from the success of preventative strategies for embolic disease in patients with atrial fibrillation, formal anticoagulation with warfarin has been suggested as a potential therapy; however, for those patients in sinus rhythm, the evidence for use of warfarin is poor. The SPIRIT study of 1997 showed that full anticoagulation of patients with previous strokes resulted in dramatically increased bleeding rates, making its use inadvisable, although less aggressive anticoagulation regimens are presently being studied.

Surgical preventative therapies in stroke disease have become increasingly prevalent following the publication of papers in 1998 demonstrating the benefits of carotid endarterectomy in symptomatic patients with significant stenosis of the common or internal carotid artery.[25] The presently accepted advice is that patients with >50 per cent stenosis and symptoms should be considered for treatment; however, despite the tenfold increased incidence of >50 per cent stenosis seen in diabetic patients compared with non-diabetic, the diabetes-related data with respect to this intervention were less clear in showing benefit, particularly in the group with 50–70 per cent stenosis, where there was no statistical outcome benefit seen with treatment, but there was a higher complications rate, especially of myocardial infarction. Thus, whilst lesions of >70 per cent stenosis are generally referred for endarterectomy, the lower grade stenoses may, as the techniques are perfected, be more appropriately treated with carotid angioplasty with stenting (in parallel to the data regarding coronary vascular disease in diabetes, where stenting has produced a much better result for diabetic patients).

7.5   Management of Acute Stroke in Diabetic Patients

The acute management of stroke concentrates on two main goals: (1) the overall supportive care and well-being of the patient; and (2) minimizing the ischaemic area of brain tissue affected by the stroke in order to maximize potential recovery.

The initial supportive care of individuals with diabetes and stroke does not differ from that of patients without diabetes who experience a stroke, and consists of basic observations and investigations to determine cause and complications.[26] Monitoring of oxygen saturation, blood pressure, pulse, temperature and respiration is vitally important, along with the provision of supplemental oxygen therapy and airway maintenance (if necessary by mechanical means). Initially oral intake should be prevented until the safety of the swallow has been assessed and assured to be stable; intravenous fluid should be commenced in order to maintain the hydration status. Diagnostic testing should include a full biochemical panel with glucose level, a full blood count, an electrocardiograph to exclude acute myocardial ischaemia (with consideration given to continuous cardiac monitoring) and an unenhanced CT scan as soon as possible. This CT scan becomes compulsory almost immediately if thrombolytic therapy is to be considered. Unless the blood pressure is severely raised, most guidelines do not recommend initial therapy for hypertension in the immediate post-stroke period, as cerebral autoregulation is usually impaired in this event and thus the ischaemic penumbra is often dependent upon systemic pressure for continued circulation. The majority of elevated blood pressure following stroke will resolve without the need for specific intervention after the first 24–48 h.

Much basic scientific work has suggested that hyperglycaemia documented in the early stages of stroke is associated with worse outcome (parallel to the observed state in cardiac disease). Hyperglycaemia is in fact a very commonly described event in acute stroke (25–50 per cent of all patients), and animal work has suggested that insulin infusions may be able to minimize the ischaemic damage from surgically induced lesions. The management of hyperglycaemia following stroke is then a common dilemma and one around which there is surprisingly little evidence or guidance. In contrast to myocardial infarction and cardiac surgery, where there has been extensive (and continued) research interest resulting in guidelines recommending glucose–insulin–potassium (GIK) infusions for acute therapy, the acute management of hyperglycaemia in stroke has not received the same attention. Whilst the practicality of GIK therapy for this group of patients has been investigated[27] and found to be feasible, there has been no study in stroke powered to determine if such therapy is beneficial to outcome, either in diabetic patients or previously non-diabetic patients with acute hypergly-caemia associated with their stroke. Indeed even the Glucose Insulin in Stroke Trial (GIST) data may not answer the feasibility question fully, as the glucose levels achieved with the infusion were not significantly different from those without the infusion. This glucose reduction in the animal data was thought to be a critical aspect of such therapies, so the real answers to this question in human stroke remain unanswered for the present. For now, then, hyperglycaemic manage-ment after stroke in clinical practice is often based on pragmatic rather than scientific principles. Known individuals with pre-existing diabetes are far more likely to receive intravenous insulin and glucose therapy than those presenting with acute hyperglycaemia; however, the duration and aggression of such therapies vary widely, and many patients receive one-off boluses of subcutaneous insulin, which is both untested and potentially more hazardous than more closely monitored intravenous therapy.

Another strategy which reflects parallel thinking to that for myocardial ischaemia is the area of thrombolysis in acute stroke. There is now significant clinical research on the practice which has demonstrated the benefits of early (<3 h from onset of symptoms) therapy with tissue-type plasminogen activator (rt-PA) for effective recovery at 3 months following ischaemic stroke, with equivalent mortality data from the two groups (an early excess of haemorrhage-associated deaths in the treated group being matched by a later excess of mortality in the untreated group).[28] Sub-analysis of diabetes patients within the study showed a greater mortality in diabetic patients, but with an equally important benefit from thrombolytic therapy. The main problem of utilizing such therapies comes from the difficulty of arranging cerebral imaging quickly enough to allow safe admin-istration of thrombolytic within the 3 h therapeutic window. This has been exemplified by the European studies[29] on the same subject using a longer treatment window (6 h), which have both been far less conclusive and which therefore leave the question of thrombolytic feasibility in Europe in question.

7.6 Diabetes and Cognitive Function

The term 'cognitive function' includes a diverse range of mental activities such as orientation, attention/concentration, perception (processing of external stimuli), memory (of all types), language, construction, reasoning, executive function (decision-making) and control of motor skills. This range includes both basic functions common to all species and most of the skills that differentiate humans from other mammals. The changes associated with diabetes in respect of cognitive functioning are relatively modest when put into this enormously wide scope; however they can be exceptionally important in the day-to-day functioning of individuals and their mood/character.

The 1990s were dubbed 'the decade of the brain' and, fittingly, it was during this decade that the associations of cognitive dysfunction and diabetes were first described in detail. Post-mortem studies had suggested that the recurrent metabolic abnormalities associated with diabetes are associated with degenerative structural change, but clinical studies had not focussed sufficiently on associating functional disturbances with this structural change. Basic clinical observation, however, had clearly described that, whilst acute hypoglycaemia is associated with pronounced cognitive impairment, acute hyperglycaemia (in the absence of acidosis or ketosis) is not. The chronic effects of hypo- or hyperglycaemia have, however, been far more difficult to determine, as experimental animal data designed to look at the problem are limited by the fact that there are clear species differences in cognitive dysfunctional processes. Thus the chronic effects of diabetes only became clear with structured and large-scale observational longitudinal studies of humans.

Acute cognitive changes

Hypoglycaemia – cognitive function and counter-regulation

The first reported cognitive changes associated with diabetes were observed during acute hypoglycaemia.[30] This observed ability to affect higher cognitive functioning was of course utilized extensively by psychiatrists in the 1950s in the form of 'insulin-shock therapy' for severe psychosis and depression. More systematic study revealed that the major effects of hypoglycaemia affected primarily the following aspects of cognition at blood sugar levels below 3 mmol/l: concentration, some aspects of memory, mental processing speed and fine motor coordination, coarse motor functions being left intact.[31] Closer study of the effects of hypoglycaemia on cognition was made possible by the use of the hyperinsulinaemic glucose clamp technique, which was extensively utilized from the 1980s in experimental study design. These studies were able to determine both the heirarchy of symptom generation from experimental hypoglycaemia and the thresholds for induction of specific cognitive dysfunction. They describe in summary:

- slowed choice-reaction times (reaction times responding to a visual stimulus with a specific action);

- slowed mental arithmetic (e.g. serial sevens);

- impaired verbal fluency (word finding);

- reduced fine manual dexterity (grooved pegboard);

- reduced hand–eye coordination;

- reduced mental flexibility (letter/number trail following tests);

- reduced story recall (long-term memory).

Occurring at blood glucose levels between 3.1 and 3.3 on average, but with considerable inter-individual variation,[32] functions such as finger tapping and other simple motor functions were barely affected. Some more subtle cognitive functions could take 60–90 min to recover after hypoglycaemia.

With such widespread cognitive effect of hypoglycaemia, it is thus unsurprising that complex day-to-day cognitive tasks (such as driving a car) are significantly impaired during acute hypoglycaemia,[33] with poor steering, road positioning, swerving and spinning when tested on driving simulators during hypoglycaemia.

One important aspect of cerebral function, which is not readily observed as an issue in fit non-diabetic individuals, but which is particularly evident when related to patients with insulin-controlled diabetes, is the control of the counter-regulatory response to hypoglycaemia itself. As blood glucose levels fall there are a number of physiological predominantly hormonal mechanisms invoked with the aim of supporting circulating glucose levels and thus maintaining cerebral (and to a lesser degree other organ) function (Figure 7.3).

In non-diabetic individuals, whilst this counter-regulatory response may be partially activated (primarily reduced insulin production with an accompanying glucagon surge) periodically in response either to starvation or prolonged physical activity, it is rarely if ever exposed to the state in which diabetic individuals may frequently find themselves, where low blood glucose levels are seen at the same time as high insulin circulating levels. Such regular triggering of the counter-regulatory response tests the physiological mechanisms to the limit, in a circumstance where the primary pancreatic counter-regulatory responses are unresponsive (the insulin levels are by definition not under counter-regulatory control, and glucagon production in response to hypoglycaemia is lost because of a failure of α/β cell communication within the islets). Thus the autonomically generated (cerebrally controlled) hormonal counter-regulatory responses are the primary form of defence from severe hypoglycaemia in diabetic individuals, and this non-physiological state can result in counter-regulatory failure and hypoglycaemia unawareness.

Encapsulating this issue is the fact that the brain is both (the most important) target organ for the adverse effects of hypoglycaemia and also the organ which is

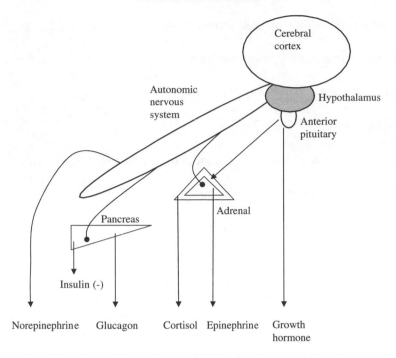

Figure 7.3 Schematic of the relationship between the hypothalamus, the pituitary and the autonomic nervous system as mediators of the counter-regulatory response

most important in controlling our metabolic responses to protect us from it. It is at risk of recurrent hypoglycaemia secondary to relative excesses in the imperfect subcutaneous route of insulin delivered in greater quantities than actually required, alternating with periods of hyperglycaemia. It has been repeatedly observed in studies using the insulin–glucose clamp technique that cerebral adaptation to repeated episodes of hypoglycaemia exists, resulting in altered (reduced) counter-regulatory hormone responses to and symptoms of hypoglycaemia. These effects result in a reduced awareness of the onset of hypoglycaemia in those frequently exposed to it. This phenomenon has been in people without diabetes (those with insulinoma) and can thus be said to represent a physiological adaptation to a non-physiological state.

Whilst the premise that adaptation to recurrent hypoglycaemia results in delayed and diminished counter-regulatory hormone responses and symptoms of acute hypoglycaemia is widely accepted, the question of higher cortical adaptation to recurrent hypoglycaemia such that global cognitive function may be better preserved during hypoglycaemia in those patients with recurrent episodes remains controversial. Some investigators have indeed found that subjects in whom counter-regulatory responses are blunted to hypoglycaemia also show preservation of cognitive function to lower glucose thresholds than patients not so adapted,[34] whilst others show deterioration of cognitive function in all subjects at consistent glucose thresholds.[35] This apparent contradiction is perhaps partly explained by the choices of cognitive function test that best represent clinically significant cerebral dysfunction during hypoglycaemia. No consensus view is held on which of the cognitive function tests used is the most significant. Some investigators prefer to use a single well-validated quick test throughout all studies (e.g. auditory or brainstem evoked potentials[36] or four-choice reaction time[37]), while others use batteries of tests, which are then analysed either singly or as a grouped 'z score'. Another confounding variable may be the duration of the hypoglycaemic stimulus. It may take a finite period of time, possibly up to 40 min, for performance to be detectably affected by the hypoglycaemia,[38] so that longer tests may be confounded. Nevertheless, the probability that different tests reflect different areas of brain with different sensitivities to hypoglycaemia is likely to underlie many of the observed discrepancies.

Investigations into the levels of glucose associated with the onset of cognitive dysfunction in individuals with delayed onset of symptomatic counter-regulatory responses to hypoglycaemia have thus been controversial. Using a summed z score technique, Mitrakou et al.[34] suggested that the blood glucose concentration for cognitive dysfunction was lower in insulinoma patients with impaired counter-regulation. Increasing latency of the P300 evoked potential (an EEG phenomenon thought to represent cortical processing of signals) associated with hypoglycaemia was also delayed in diabetic subjects with hypoglycaemia unawareness.[39] In normal subjects studied after 56 h of enforced moderate hypoglycaemia (2.9 mmol/l), Boyle et al.[40] demonstrated preservation of performance in Stroop tests and finger tapping to lower glucose levels, associated with better preservation of cerebral glucose uptake and delayed counter-regulation. These data suggest a *global* adaptation of the human brain to preceding hypoglycaemia, involving both glucose sensing regions and the cerebral cortex. One possible mechanism is a hypoglycaemia-induced up-regulation of endothelial glucose transporters.

However, the clinical picture of defective symptomatic counter-regulatory responses, hypoglycaemia unawareness and increased risk of severe hypoglycaemia (summarized figuratively in Figure 7.4) does not fit with such global adaptive change and clinically suggests the experimentally supported notion that there is no preservation of cognitive function during hypoglycaemia in hypoglycaemia-prone diabetic patients, despite substantial delay in the onset of counter-regulatory responses. Several investigators have described dissociation between the onset of counter-regulatory responses and cognitive dysfunction during acute hypoglycaemia in patients with diabetes,[35] suggesting that the degree of adaptation of cerebral response to hypoglycaemia may vary regionally throughout the brain. Thus, whilst the deleterious effects of hypoglycaemia on cortical cerebral function remain relatively unchanged whatever the previous experience of hypoglycaemia, the effectiveness of the counter-regulatory response may vary widely depending on previous experience of hypoglycaemia. This is described in the model proposed in

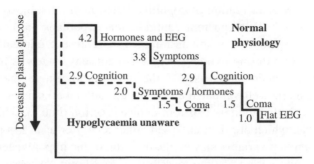

Figure 7.4 Schematic representation of glycaemic thresholds for change associated with hypoglycaemia. The solid line represents thresholds for change in normal physiology, whilst the dashed line represents individuals exposed to frequent hypoglycaemia with regional adaptation, resulting in hypoglycaemia unawareness, as cognitive function is impaired before any symptom generation

1992 by Philip Cryer, which he termed 'hypoglycaemia-associated autonomic failure', bringing together in a single model all the aspects associated with cerebral function described in Figure 7.1.[41]

The exact cortical mechanisms underlying the triggering of counter-regulation remain under intense investigational scrutiny, with recent studies concentrating on regional rates of change in cerebral glucose metabolism (particularly in the ventromedial nucleus of the hypothalamus)[42] as a likely, although not yet definitively proven, source. However, despite this uncertainty in the basic physiology, there are a number of clearly observed clinical phenomena which are able to inform the management of patients with hypoglycaemia unawareness with its concomitant increased risk of severe hypoglycaemia. Developing observations made after the successful removal of insulinomas and the effects seen on the normalization of previously abnormal counter-regulation, three separate groups of researchers observed that the strict avoidance of hypoglycaemia in day-to-day life will result in improvement towards normal of the counter-regulatory hormonal response where it has previously been blunted, regained awareness of warning symptoms for hypoglycaemia and reduced risk of severe hypoglycaemia.[35,43,44] This is encouraging research data, particularly as the researchers in closely supervised day-to-day activity were able to achieve avoidance of hypoglycaemia without significant deterioration of overall control (and indeed in some individuals with particularly fluctuant control even an improvement in HbA1c). However, the amount of clinical input required in these studies (and indeed in those DCCT centres where improved glycaemic control was achieved without increasing the risk of incident hypoglycaemia) is perhaps at a higher level that is practical in the normal day-to-day clinical care for the vast majority of our patients; thus it is important to look for the key clinical interventions that seem to have the most impact on hypoglycaemia avoidance.

(1) *Insulin regimens* – over the last decade much attention has been paid to the development of analogue insulins which might be able to mimic more closely the 'physiological' insulin secretion curve and thus reduce the periods when individuals are exposed in inappropriate hyper- or hypoinsulinaemia, with resultant glucose fluctuations. Within the confines of closely regulated studies, some significant success has been achieved both with short-acting (prandial) insulin analogues (e.g. Humalog and Novorapid), which (with judicious and appropriate use) reduce the pre-meal exposure to hyperinsulinaemia, and long-acting (basal) analogues (e.g. Glargine and Detemir), which can reduce the overnight exposure to hyperinsulinaemia at a time when physiologically the insulin secretion levels are very low. The most successful insulin regimen in studies for the avoidance of hypoglycaemia in well-motivated patients is, however, clearly the use of continuous subcutaneous insulin infusions (CSII) which, because of the ability to adjust basal infusion rates across the day and to infuse very small boluses frequently if so required, along with the fact that the subcutaneous 'insulin reservoir' at any given time is very small (thus resulting in more predictable absorption), provides for very precise insulin adjustment in those who monitor their glucose levels sufficiently closely to allow it. However, despite these advances, the type of insulin or method of injection will not allow hypoglycaemia avoidance reliably if used in isolation of other (often more important) aspects of daily life, or in those people whose attention to glucose fluctuations is less close than individuals used in studies.

(2) *Physical activity* is clearly an important part of daily routine to which attention must be addressed if hypoglycaemia is to be avoided. The type, intensity, duration and timing of exercise along with the conditions in which it is conducted (ambient temperature, underlying fitness of the individual, etc.) will all impact on the glycaemic excursion seen during and after a bout of activity. Thus, if hypoglycaemia is a problem, then activity and insulin/carbohydrate responses to it need to be carefully planned in advance with knowledge of the individual and their insulin sensitivity as an integral part of such planning. This is an often ignored aspect of day-to-day glucose control, especially for unplanned bouts of activity (e.g. sex), on which attention deserves to be more focussed in the future.

(3) *Diet*, like activity, is obviously an important determinant of glucose excursions, particularly the carbohydrate component of diet. It is increasingly being recognised that the day-to-day variations in both the size and content of a normal healthy diet require both knowledge of glycaemic effect and planning in order to minimize glucose excursion, especially if hypoglycaemia is a problem. 'Carbohydrate counting' (usually in 10 g portions) with knowledge of the carbohydrate–insulin ratio (traditionally expressed as units of insulin per 10 g carbohydrate portion) is a basic necessity if such glucose excursions

are to be minimized, but additionally glycaemic index, glycaemic load and meal composition will all have significant impacts and require attention. Additionally the timing of carbohydrate intake is an important consideration in the overall glucose control over 24 h, particularly in the form of between-meal snacks for those individuals who, based on previous experience, have a reproducible time when the risk of hypoglycaemia is greatest.

(4) *'Awareness training' and continuous monitoring* – symptomatic awareness of hypoglycaemia relies both on the generation of symptoms and the correct recognition of those symptoms as a feature of impending hypoglycaemia. Over time the symptoms generated may change so that individuals fail to recognize them even when they are present. There has been some success using biofeedback techniques to improve recognition of symptoms earlier in the fall of glucose, especially when the symptoms may be idiosyncratic or atypical and otherwise missed. The appropriate use of finger-stick monitoring is clearly important for hypoglycaemia avoidance during the day, but in addition to the goal-orientated use of such monitoring, the more detailed 'minimally invasive' continuous monitoring techniques based upon continuous subcutaneous sampling techniques have over the course of the last decade significantly improved the recognition of hypoglycaemia risk periods, especially when those periods occur at night when the individual would otherwise be unaware of them. Indeed one of the major causes of hypoglycaemia unawareness may be following recurrent unidentified nocturnal hypoglycaemic exposure with no clearly identifiable pattern of recurrent daytime hypoglycaemic experience.

(5) *Education programmes*, based upon the pioneering work of Michael Berger and the Düsseldorf group – there has been increasing recognition worldwide over the last decade of the importance of the patient as the expert in self-management, particularly where issues of day-to-day control are involved. Additionally, the traditional educational process of group learning has finally been successfully incorporated into the routine clinical practice of diabetes education with significant impact for the psychological and physical health of individuals with diabetes. Glycaemia management and hypoglycaemia avoidance form the mainstay of many of these programmes, such as the recently studied DAFNE (Dose Adjustment For Normal Eating) programme in the UK.

(6) *Drugs* – whilst a pharmaceutical product to allow continued timely recognition of hypoglycaemia has not been identified, many substances have been shown to have modulatory effects upon glycaemia awareness, and the search for appropriate pharmacological intervention continues to gather pace, encouraged by experimental data using such 'everyday' compounds such as

caffeine. In studies of hypoglycaemia, it has been found that prior dosing with caffeine enhances hypoglycaemic awareness – albeit to a relatively mild degree.

Chronic cognitive changes and diabetes

In addition to the excess risk of vascular disease occurring in diabetic subjects (discussed previously), the epidemiology of cognitive impairment has reliably shown a link between type 2 diabetes and the risk of accelerated cognitive decline.[45] Although the nature of this association was initially unclear, more recent data suggest that there is a significant relationship between cognitive decline and levels of glucose control in diabetes which may be ameliorated by improved glucose control in line with other diabetes-related complications.[46] Further, there have been independent studies looking at the frequency of Alzheimer's disease in the population which also describe a clear relationship between it and diabetes, thus there are a number of different issues in the development of chronic cognitive change in individuals with diabetes, addressed below.

Hypoglycaemia-related chronic cognitive dysfunction

Following hypoglycaemic coma, recovery of neurological function is usually rapid with no discernable cognitive effect after 36 h. However, a single episode of severe hypoglycaemia, if coma is protracted, can (rarely) result in permanent neurological dysfunction and structural abnormality, with lesions described predominantly in the frontal areas and deep grey matter. Such lesions are rarely encountered in day-to-day practice. The more common clinical picture of recurrent variable hypoglycaemia over many years has a more uncertain impact upon cognitive function. Most investigators fail to determine any specific detriment of such experience when studying its effect in adults, but occasional reports of predisposition to later life cognitive decline and cortical atrophy have been documented. Perhaps the most complete documentation of such risk[47] was made in 2003 in a group of 74 young adults with type 1 diabetes (all >10 years' duration), in whom a cognitive battery of tests was undertaken, along with an MRI, and analysed according to prior hypoglycaemic experience (total severe hypoglycaemic episodes) and evidence of retinopathy as a marker for hyperglycaemia. In this study hypoglycaemic experience had no detectable deleterious long-term effect on either cognitive function or brain structure, whilst the group with retinopathy had significant impairments of aspects of cognitive function and small focal white matter lesions in the basal ganglia. Data for hypoglycaemic effects in children are equally reassuring, except for those who develop diabetes very early in life (<5 years old), in whom severe hypoglycaemia at such a young age appears to have a significant (if relatively small) effect on later measures of intelligence.

Ischaemia-related cognitive decline

As described earlier in this chapter, type 2 diabetes is associated with an increased risk of stroke, and whilst large infarctive events clearly have significant impact upon an individual's cognition, population studies have additionally described increased cortical atrophy occurring in diabetic patients without focal lesions,[48] which are postulated to be either a microangiopathic effect of diabetes or multiple small macrovascular disease-mediated infarcts possibly related to hypertension or the effects of other metabolic derangement occurring in patients with poorly controlled diabetes such as uraemia with 'middle molecule'-mediated cognitive decline. Conclusive data is, however, not yet available as, while studies of cognitive decline with age in diabetes have been undertaken,[49] and neuroimaging studies with large numbers of patients have also been described, there is not yet a large study that has combined both these measurements in the same population. However, MRI studies have also identified white matter hyperintensities (leukoaraiosis), which are felt to represent 'ischaemic demyelination' secondary to occlusion of small penetrating arteries. Further, the frequency of such lesions is associated with the level of glycaemic control over time.[48] More recent and more detailed gadolinium-enhanced MRI investigation of diabetic volunteers compared with non-diabetic subjects has revealed increased blood–brain barrier permeability in patients with diabetes and white matter lesions,[50] suggesting that this may reflect one of the underlying causes of cerebral dysfunction in patients with diabetes and potentially other conditions similarly affecting the brain, such as hypertension.

In terms of frequency it is likely that such vascular-mediated cerebral changes are the most important cause of the amplified cognitive decline over time seen in patients with diabetes (both type 1[51] and type 2[49]) as compared with the population without diabetes. In this recently opened field of investigation, however, there are other possibilities for the cause of such decline, so that definitive statements regarding the relative importance of different causes will require further study for clarification.

Diabetes and Alzheimer's disease

As both diabetes and Alzheimer's disease tend to occur in older populations, the association between the two conditions was for many years felt to be purely coincidental. However, recent studies[52] into the association have clearly identified that there is indeed a link that is more powerful than chance alone (although no causality can be at this stage implied). One recent longitudinal study[52] looked at an ageing population of nuns and priests, following them both with cognitive function testing and formal examinations for the development of Alzheimers disease. Those of the population with diabetes had a 65 per cent increase in the risk of developing

Alzheimer's disease (based upon international diagnostic guidelines) over 5 years and a 44 per cent increase in the speed of cognitive decline overall. In addition to such clinical data, imaging studies[53] revealed a characteristic early effect on the hippocampus and amygdale in patients with Alzheimer's disease. A recent large population study of MRI imaging in elderly subjects (>500 individuals) with and without diabetes showed more atrophy in the diabetic subjects that the non-diabetic, with the greatest atrophy seen in those with the highest levels of insulin resistance, and occurring independent of any vascular abnormalities.[53] Although there is not yet any human post-mortem study showing the characteristic neuropathological changes of Alzheimer's disease associated with diabetes (which would obviously clinch the case), there is now experimental animal evidence which has found characteristic Alzheimer-type change in animals exposed to hyperglycaemia over time. At this stage, then (although the cause of the link is unclear), one can reliably state that the risk of Alzheimer's disease is indeed elevated in diabetes. Interestingly, there has also been work reported looking at the glucose metabolic status of patients with Alzheimers disease, which would tend to suggest that diabetes is more common in this group than in the comparable age–sex-matched population with dementia of non-Alzheimer type.[54] This study did involve some autopsy studies and made the link between Alzheimer's and type 2 diabetes on the basis of amyloid beta protein deposition occurring in the brain in Alzheimer's and the pancreas in type 2 diabetes as a possible unifying source of causation.

Diabetes and psychiatric disease

Any discussion of the central nervous system and diabetes would not be complete without reference to the long-described association between diabetes and psychiatric disease. In recent years the focus for clinicians managing glucose abnormalities in patients with psychiatric disease has focussed on the case reports (including fatalities) of new-onset diabetes and hyperglycaemic emergencies associated with the use of atypical antipsychotic drugs. This is, however, whilst important as a clinical risk, almost certainly a mis-representation of the overall relationship between glucose metabolism and patients with psychiatric illness, and indeed mimics the spate of similar reports in the early 1950s when the first antipsychotic agent (chlorpromazine) became available. Following initial associative observations as early as 1897 – 'Diabetes is a disease which often shows itself in families where insanity prevails' (Henry Maudsley) – for over 60 years the excess incidence of type 2 diabetes and the metabolic syndrome has been noted, particularly in association with schizophrenia. This association has thus been made for longer than there have been antipsychotic medications available and it seems likely from more recent controlled studies[55] that glucose intolerance and diabetes are inherent aspects of schizophrenia (perhaps relating to chronic 'stress' activation of the sympathoadrenal–medullary and hypothalamic–pituitary–adrenal axes, resulting in excess secretion of epinephrine, norepinephrine and cortisol), which may be exacerbated by lifestyle changes associated with psychiatric disease and further by the drugs used to treat psychiatric illness. Thus, although it is probably multifactorial, it would seem that the most powerful link between the cognitive dysfunction associated with psychiatric disease and diabetes is mediated via insulin resistance. Indeed the Food and Drug Administration in the United States recommends that all patients with schizophrenia (particularly if to be treated with antipsychotic agents) should be screened for glucose intolerance and diabetes.[56]

7.7 Summary

It is perhaps to be expected that the brain, as an organ exclusively dependent upon the supply of glucose for its continuing functions, and supplied with a rich vascular tree for this purpose, can have its function dramatically influenced in a condition which changes those glucose levels, and exposes individuals to a wide (non-physiological) range of glycaemic experience from episodic hypoglycaemia to chronic hyperglycaemia. All aspects of the complex interplay of modulators (Figure 7.1), which produces the unique cognitive outcomes of personality, character and and intelligence that characterize individuals, can be affected by the consequences of diabetes (either directly or indirectly). The majority of such effects have only been systematically investigated in the course of the last decade or so, such that the present state of knowledge is really only scratching the surface of the issues. However, now that some of the more important issues have been brought into the spotlight, and many of the the the underlying cerebral mechanisms are being elucidated,[57] the next decade should, based upon the increasing awareness of the cerebral molecular changes associated with diabetes, start to yield not just new descriptions of problems, but the hope for answers to the issues of defective cognitive and cerebral function that can accompany diabetes.

References

1. Hankey GJ. Stroke: how large a public health problem and how can the neurologist help? *Arch Neurol* 1999; **56**: 748–754.
2. Currie CJ, Morgan CL, Gill L, Scott NCH, Peters JR. Epidemiology and cost of acute hospital care for cerebrovascular disease in diabetic and non-diabetic populations. *Stroke* 1997; **28**: 1142–1146.
3. Aronson SM. Intracranial vascular lesions in patients with diabetes mellitus. *J Neuropathol Exp Neurol* 1973; **32**: 183–196.
4. Deckert T, Poulsen JE, Larsen M. Prognosis of diabetics with diabetes onset before the age of 31. I. Survival, causes of death and complications. *Diabetologia* 1978; **14**: 363–370.

5. Pulsinelli W, Levy DE, Sigsbee B, Scherer P, Plum F. Increased damage after ischaemic stroke in patients with hyperglycaemia with or without established diabetes mellitus. *Am J Med* 1983; **74**: 540–543.

6. Capes SE. How critical is blood glucose to the outcome of stroke? *Neurol Rev* 1999; **7**: 26–30.

7. Davis TME, Millns H, Stratton IM, Holman RR, Turner RC. Risk factors for stroke in type 2 diabetes mellitus: United Kingdom Prospective Diabetes Study (UKPDS) 29. *Arch Intern Med* 1999; **159**: 1097–1103.

8. Williams B, Poulter NR, Brown MJ, Davis M, McInnes GT, Potter JF, Sever PS, Thom SM. British Hypertension Society Guidelines for hypertension management 2004 (BHS-IV): summary. *Br Med J* 2004; **328**: 634–640.

9. Stroke Prevention in AF investigators. Adjusted dose warfarin versus low intensity fixed dose warfarin plus aspirin for high risk patients with non-valvular atrial fibrillation. *Lancet* 1996; **348**: 633–638.

10. Sacco RL, Foulkes MA, Mohr JP, Worf PA, Hier DB, Price TR. Determinants of early recurrence of cerebral infarction: the stroke data bank. *Stroke* 1989; **20**: 983–989.

11. Petty GW, Brown RD, Whisnant JP, Sicks JD, O'Fallon WM, Wiebers DO. Survival and recurrence after first cerebral infarction: a population-based study in Rochester, Minnesota, 1975–1989. *Neurology* 1998; **50**: 208–216.

12. Lai SM, Alter M, Firday G, Sobel E. A multifactorial analysis of risk-factors for recurrence of ischaemic stroke. *Stroke* 1994; **25**: 958–962.

13. Scandinavian Simvastatin Survival Group. Randomised trial of cholesterol lowering in 4444 patients with coronary artery disease: the Scandinavian Simvastatin Survival Study (4S). *Lancet* 1994; **344**: 1383–1389.

14. Pyorala K, Pedersen TR, Kjekshus J, Faergeman O, Olsson AG, Thorgeirsson G. Cholseterol lowering with simvastatin improves the prognosis of diabetic patients with coronary heart disease. *Diabetes Care* 1997; **20**(4): 614–620.

15. Law MR, Wald NJ, Rudnicka AR. Quantifying effect of statins on low density lipoprotein cholesterol, ischaemic heart disease, and stroke: systematic review and meta-analysis. *Br Med J* 2003; **326**: 1423–1429.

16. Collins R, Armitage J, Parish S, Sleight P, Peto R. Heart Protection Study Collaborative Group. Effects of cholesterol-lowering with simvastatin on stroke and other major vascular events in 20536 people with cerebrovascular disease or other high-risk conditions. *Lancet* 2004; **363**(9411): 757–767.

17. The Heart Outcomes Prevention Evaluation(HOPE) Study Investigators. Effects of ramipril on cardiovascular and microvascular outcomes in people with diabetes mellitus: results of Hope study and MICRO-HOPE substudy. *Lancet* 2000; **355**: 253–259.

18. PROGRESS Collaborative Group (writing committee: MacMahon S, Neal B, Tzourio C, Rodgers A, Woodward M, Cutler J, Anderson C and Chalmers J with the assistance of Ohkubo T). Randomised trial of a perindopril-based blood pressure lowering regimen among 6,105 individuals with previous stroke or transient ischaemic attack. *Lancet* 2001; **358**: 1033–1041.

19. PROGRESS Collaborative Group (writing committee: Tzourio C, Anderson C, Chapman N, Woodward M, Neal N, MacMahon S, Chalmers J). Effects of blood pressure lowering with perindopril and indapamide on dementia and cognitive decline in patients with cerebrovascular disease. *Arch Intern Med* 2003; **163**: 1069–1075.

20. PROGRESS Collaborative Group (writing committee: Fransen M, Anderson C, Chalmers J, Chapman N, Davis S, MacMahon S, Neal B, Sega R, Trent A, Tzourio C, Woodward M). The effects of a perindopril-based blood pressure lowering regimen on disability and dependency in 6,105 patients with cerebrovascular disease. A randomised controlled trial. *Stroke* 2003; **34**: 2333–2338.

21. Antiplatelet Triallists Collaboration. Collaborative overview of randomised trials of anti-platelet therapy. 1. Prevention of death, myocardial infarction and stroke by prolonged antiplatelet therapy in various categories of patients. *Br Med J* 1994; **308**: 81–106.

22. CAPRIE Steering Committee. A randomised blinded trial of clopidogrel versus aspirin in patients at risk of ischaemic events. *Lancet* 1996; **348**: 1329–1339.

23. Ringleb PA, Bhatt DL, Hirsh AT, Topol EJ, Hacke W. Benefit of Clopidogrel over aspirin is amplified in patients with a history of ischaemic events. *Stroke* 2004; **35**: 528–532.

24. Diener HC, Chnha L, Forbes J, Sivenius P, Smets P, Lowenthal A. European Stroke Prevention Study 2. Dipyridamole and acetylsalicylic acid in the secondary prevention of stroke. *J Neurol Sci* 1996; **143**: 1–13.

25. European Carotid Surgery Triallists Collaborative Group. Randomised trial of endarter-ectomy for recently symptomatic carotid stenoses: final results of the MRC European Carotid Surgery Trail. *Lancet* 1998; **351**: 1379–1387.

26. Intercollegiate Stroke Working Party. *National Guidelines for Stroke*, 2nd edn. Royal College of Physicians: London, 2004; available at www.rcplondon.ac.uk (accessed 14 April 2005).

27. Scott JF, Robinson GM, French JM, O'Connell JE, Alberti KGMM, Gray CS. Glucose Potassium Insulin Infusions in the treatment of acute strokepatients with mild to moderate hyperglycaemia. The Glucose Insulin in Stroke Trial (GIST). *Stroke* 1999; **39**: 793–799.

28. The National Institute of Neurologic Disorders and *Stroke* (NINDS) rt-PA Stroke Study Group. Tissue plasminogen activator for acute ischaemic stroke. *New Engl J Med* 1995; **333**: 1581–1587.

29. The European Co-operative Acute Stroke Study (ECASS). Intravenous thrombolysis with recombinant tissue plasminogen activator for acute hemispheric stroke. *JAMA* 1995; **274**: 1017–1025.

30. Fletcher AA, Campbell WR. The blood sugar following insulin administration and the symptom complex – hypoglycaemia. *J Metab Res* 1922; **2**: 637–649.

31. Russell PN, Rix-Trot HM. An exploratory study of some behavioural consequences of insulin-induced hypoglycaemia. *NZ Med J* 1975; **81**: 337–340.

32. Deary IJ. The effects of hypoglycaemia on cognitive function. In Frier BM and Fisher BM (eds), *Hypoglycaemia in Diabetes: Clinical and Physiological Aspects*. London: Edward Arnold, 1993; 80–92.

33. Cox DJ, Gonder-Frederick LA, Clark W. Driving decrements in type 1 diabetes during moderate hypoglycaemia. *Diabetes* 1993; **42**: 239–243.

34. Mitrakou A, Fanelli C, Veneman T, Perriello G, Calderone S, Platanisiotis D, Rambotti A, Raptis S, Brunetti, P, Cryer P, Gerich J, Bolli G. Reversibilty of unawareness of hypogly-caemia in patients with insulinomas. *New Engl J Med* 1993; **329**: 834–839.

35. Cranston I, Lomas J, Maran A, Macdonald I, Amiel SA. Restoration of hypoglycaemia awareness in patients with long-duration insulin-dependent diabetes. *Lancet* 1994; **344**: 283–287.

36. Martini A, Comacchio F, Magnavita V. Auditory brainstem and middle latency evoked responses in the clinical evaluation of diabetes. *Diab Med* 1991; **8**: S74–77.

37. Wilkinson RT, Houghton D. Portable four-choice reaction time test with magnetic tape memory. *Behav Res Meth Instrum* 1975; **7**: 441–446.

38. Kerr D, Macdonald IA, Tattersall RB. Patients with type 1 diabetes adapt acutely to sustained mild hypoglycaemia. *Diabet Med* 1991; **8**: 123–128.

39. Zeigler D, Hubinger A, Muhlers H, Gries FA. Effect of previous glycaemic control on the onset and the magnitude of cognitive dysfunction during hypoglycaemia in Type one diabetic patients. *Diabetologia* 1992; **35**: 828–834.

40. Boyle PJ, Nagy RJ, O'Connor AM, Kempers SF, Yeo RA, Qualls C. Adaptation in brain glucose uptake following recurrent hypoglycemia. *Proc Nat Acad Sci USA* 1994; **91**: 9352–9356.

41. Cryer PE, Davis SN, Shamoon H. Hypoglycaemia in diabetes. *Diabet Care* 2003; **26**: 1902–1912.

42. Cranston IC, Reed LJ, Marsden PK, Amiel SA. Changes in regional brain ^{18}F-fluoro-deoxyglucose uptake at hypoglycaemia in type 1 diabetic men associated with hypoglycaemia unawareness and counter-regulatory failure. *Diabetes* 2001; **50**: 2329–2336.

43. Fanelli CG, Epifano L, Rambotti AM, Pampanelli S, Di Vincenzo A, Modarelli F, Lepore M, Annibqle B, Ciofetta M, Bottini P, Porcellati F, Scionti L, Santeusanio F, Brunetti P, Bolli GB. Meticulous prevention of hypoglycemia normalises glycemic thresholds and magnitude of most of the neuroendocrine responses to, and symptoms of, and cognitive function during hypoglcyemia in intensively-treated patients with short-term IDDM. *Diabetes* 1993; **42**: 1683–1689.

44. Dagogo-Jack S, Rattarasarn C, Cryer PE. Reversal of hypoglycemia unawareness, but not defective glucose counter-regulation, in IDDM. *Diabetes* 1994; **43**: 1426–1434.

45. Richardson JT. Cognitive function in diabetes. *Neurosci Behav Rev* 1990; **14**(4): 385–388.

46. Greenwood CE, Kaplan RJ, Hebblethwaite S, Jenkins DJA. Carbohydrate-Induced memory impairment in adults with type 2 diabetes. *Diabet Care* 2003; **26**: 1961–1966.

47. Ferguson SC, Blane A, Perros P, McCrimmon RJ, Best JK, Wardlaw J, Deary IJ, Frier BM. Cognitive ability and brain structure in type 1 diabetes, relation to microangiopathy and preceding severe hypoglycaemia. *Diabetes* 2003; **52**: 149–156.

48. Schmidt R, Launer LJ, Nilsson LG, Pajak A, Sans S, Berger K, Breteler MM, de Ridder M, Dufouil C, Fuhres R, Giampaoli S, Hofman A for the CASCADE consortium. Magnetic resonance imaging of the brain in diabetes – the cardiovascular determinants of dementia (CASCADE) study. *Diabetes* 2004; **53**: 687–692.

49. Logroscino G, Kang JH, Grodstein F. Prospective study of type 2 diabetes and cognitive decline in women aged 70–81 yrs. *Br Med J* 2004; **328**(7439): 548.

50. Starr JM, Wardlaw J, Ferguson K, MacLullich A, Deary IJ, Marshall I. Increased blood–brain barrier permeability in type 2 diabetes demonstrated by gadolinium magnetic resonance imaging. *J Neurol Neurosug Psychiat* 2003; **74**: 70–76.

51. Ryan CM, Geckle MO, Orchard TJ. Cognitive efficiency declines over time in adults with type 1 diabetes: effects of micro- and macrovascular complications. *Diabetologia* 2003; **46**: 940–948.

52. Arvanitakis Z, Wilson RS, Bienas JL, Evans DA, Bennett DA. Diabetes mellitus and the risk of Alzheimer's disease and decline in cognitive function. *Arch Neurol* 2004; **61**: 661–666.

53. Den Heijer T, Vermeer SE, van Dijk EJ, Prins ND, Koudstaal PJ, Hofman A. type 2 diabetes and atrophy of medial temporal lobe structures on brain MRI. *Diabetologia* 2003; **46**: 1604–1610.

54. Janson J, Laedtke T, Parisi JE, O'Brien P, Petersen RC, Butler PC. Increased risk of type 2 diabetes in Alzheimer disease. *Diabetes* 2004; **53**: 474–481.

55. Ryan MC, Collins P, Thakore JH. Impaired fasting glucose tolerance in first-episode, drug-naïve patients with schizophrenia. *Am J Psychiat* 2003; **160**: 284–289.

56. American Diabetes Association, American Psychiatric Association, American Association of Clinical Endocrinologists, North American Association for the Study of Obesity. Consensus development conference on antipsychotic drugs and obesity and diabetes. *Diabet Care* 2004; **27**(2): 596–601.

57. Klein JP, Waxman SG. The brain in diabetes: molecular changes in neurons and their implications for end-organ damage. *Lancet Neurol* 2003; **2**: 548–554.

8

Diabetes and the Gastrointestinal System

Charles Murray and **Anton Emmanuel**

8.1 Introduction

For many years it was felt that the prevalence of gastrointestinal (GI) symptoms in the diabetic population was not greater than that in the general population. Over the last 10–15 years, however, advances in our understanding of GI physiology and classification of symptoms have revealed that diabetic patients do in fact have a large burden of GI symptoms and that this is associated with sensory and motor GI abnormalities. The identification of gastrointestinal symptoms attributable to diabetes remains a challenge. For example, the gut is a neurally complex organ with as many neurones in the enteric nervous system as the spinal cord. If we consider that many diabetic complications described elsewhere in the body are secondary to neuropathy, then it would appear intuitive that diabetes could affect GI function at multiple different levels.

Historically, the only major GI symptom associated with diabetes was intractable vomiting, ascribed physiologically to delayed gastric emptying or gastroparesis. The association of diabetes mellitus with delayed gastric emptying was described as long ago as 1925 by Boas,[1] and 30 years later Kassander termed the condition 'gastroparesis diabeticorum', a term which has survived to the present day.[2] Gastroparesis remains a difficult problem to treat (see below), but in addition it is clear that diabetes can affect the whole GI tract. Having said this, it would be wrong to ascribe all GI symptoms as secondary to diabetes without excluding other causes, and the work-up of these patients should still involve a full medical history

Diabetes: Chronic Complications Edited by Kenneth M. Shaw and Michael H. Cummings
© 2005 John Wiley & Sons, Ltd.

and examination followed by the pertinent investigations as one would for a non-diabetic patient with GI symptoms.

In this chapter we will discuss each part of the GI tract systematically and explain the symptoms and pathophysiological abnormalities that can be associated with diabetes. For each symptom complex we will summarize the screening and investigation process and the subsequent management of these patients.

8.2 Epidemiology

Although we have a better understanding of the effects of diabetes on the gut, there remains some controversy in the literature as to the extent to which patients with diabetes complain of gastrointestinal symptoms. Most studies have focused on tertiary referral groups, and it is not until recently that large community-based studies have given us a truer idea of prevalence.[3] Studies range from those reporting large increases in the prevalence of upper GI symptoms only[4] to those showing no difference between patients and controls,[5] to others reporting increased frequency of all GI symptoms in diabetic patients.[4,6-9] Some studies report duration of disease as an independent factor associated with GI symptoms,[7] while other studies have not observed this association.[3] It had formally been assumed that GI symptoms are secondary to autonomic neuropathy affecting the gut.[10,11] Indeed, cardiovascular autonomic neuropathy has been correlated with oesophageal dysmotility, gastroparesis, heartburn, dyspepsia, constipation, diarrhoea and incontinence in patients with diabetes mellitus. However, in the majority of cases it does not appear that autonomic neuropathy is the primary cause, since large-scale epidemiological studies have shown no correlation between symptoms and neuropathy.[12] An alternative pathophysiological factor could be hyperglycaemia, which on its own can cause gut dysfunction at any level of the gastrointestinal tract.[13-16] Furthermore, it would appear that the actual level of blood glucose has significant correlation with gut symptoms.[3]

What these studies point out is that a number of factors contribute to the development of gut symptoms in patients with diabetes. Certainly, the role of tight blood sugar control should be emphasized (as with prevention of other complications). This is both in terms of primary prevention and in terms of acute symptom control, since hyperglycaemia has acute physiological effects on the whole GI tract (see below). The duration of diabetes may also be important as well as any other associated autonomic neuropathy. However, larger population studies are needed, and until recently have been hampered by the lack of consistency in the instrument used to collect data, something that may now be improved by the development of the Diabetes Bowel Symptom Questionnaire.[17] What is clear form the literature is that, regardless of site of symptomatology and which factors are associated with these gut symptoms, their presence leads to a significant impairment of the quality of life of diabetic patients.[18]

8.3 Pathophysiology of GI Dysfunction

Neuropathy

Investigators have found abnormalities at a number of different neurological levels in diabetic patients. Gastroparesis represents the paradigm condition of diabetic involvement of the gut and is the most studied condition. It was initially felt that the majority of detrimental effects of diabetes on the gut were secondary to vagal neuropathy, since the effects of vagotomy appeared very similar to the physiological findings in patients with gastroparesis. However, while this may be relevant in some symptomatic patients, it is not ubiquitously present. Abnormalities are present in both the parasympathetic and sympathetic autonomic systems in gastroparetic patients, and additionally there are enteric nervous system abnormalities. These will be discussed with respect to specific GI systems, but first it is important to summarize some of these abnormalities, since they will be relevant to subsequent management and treatment strategies.

Level of abnormality

Diabetic autonomic neuropathy is a common and serious complication of diabetes, which can involve the entire autonomic nervous system (ANS), significantly impairing the survival and quality of life of diabetic patients. Most studies find that the presence of cardiac autonomic neuropathy leads to an increased relative risk of death within a 5 year period, the highest reported relative risk being 9.2.[19] There are many possible explanations of this phenomenon, including a metabolic insult to nerve fibres, neurovascular insufficiency, autoimmune damage and neurohumoral growth factor deficiency.[20] As well as multiple possible aetiologies to this neuropathy, there are also multiple levels at which this neuropathy could affect bowel function.

Enteric abnormalities

There has been much speculation as to the role of intrinsic enteric neuropathy in diabetics. A histological silver staining technique to evaluate the myenteric plexus showed these nerves to be nomal in patients with diabetes.[21] In contrast Burnstock and colleagues have documented disturbances in intrinsic nerves and the protective role of gangliosides in a series of studies in the streptozotocin rat model of diabetes.[22–26] They have shown a deficiency of nitrergic neurons in the pyloric sphincter as well as a decrease in inhibitory neurotransmitters and an increase in excitatory transmitters in non-sphincteric muscle. Additionally, two recent studies have also demonstrated abnormalities in the pacemaker cells of the upper gut. In an animal study, Ordog *et al.*[27] have shown electrophysiological disturbances associated with reduced volume of the pacemaker cells in the gut, interstitial cells of Cajal (ICC), in the gastric antrum and fundus. A single case study from the Cleveland and Mayo clinic showed a reduced ICC network in the jejunum in a diabetic patient, and this was associated with reduced numbers of neurons staining for neuronal nitric oxide synthase (nNOS) and vasoactive intestinal polypeptide (VIP).[28] Low levels of nNOS have previously been reported in animal models of diabetes, an abnormality that is reversed by insulin.[29]

Both these studies have shown a decrease in number and remodelling of interstitial cells of Cajal. The patients study also showed a decrease in inhibitory innervation at an enteric nervous system level with an associated increase in excitatory innervation. Hence abnormalities at an enteric nervous system level will certainly have a role to play.

Autonomic abnormalities

It has long been recognized that gastroparetic patients have vagal dysfunction,[30] and several of the motor abnormalities observed in symptomatic diabetic patients are indistinguishable from those seen in patients with other syndromes that affect postganglionic sympathetic function.[31] Differences found in the lower gut of diabetic patients are thought to be secondary to neuropathic rather than myopathic factors, since the effect of direct smooth muscle stimulation is the same in both diabetics and healthy controls.[32] In a rat model of diabetic diarrhoea, α_2-adrenergic tone is impaired,[33] and it is thought that this in turn leads to impaired water and electrolyte transport, hence resulting in diarrhoea.

The degree to which gut neuropathy is associated with cardiac autonomic neuropathy (CAN) is not clear. The reported prevalence of the latter varies considerably depending on how CAN is defined and the population being studied. For example, a community-based study of diabetic neuropathy in Oxford has reported a prevalence of 16.7 per cent,[34] compared with another multicentre study, which reported a prevalence of 25.3 per cent in type I diabetics and 34.3 per cent in type II diabetics.[35] Determination of gut-specific neuropathy in these patients has been difficult up to now due to insufficient tools to measure gut-specific autonomic outflow. Evolving techniques of studying enteric neurophysiology, gut-specific autonomic function and central nerve activation afford the opportunity of advancing our ability to classify these symptom complexes in a physiological framework.[36,37]

Central abnormalities

There is an evolving understanding of the importance of central processing in other functional gut disorders, and it is likely that this is important in the pathophysiology of diabetic gut symptoms. Recent functional imaging studies have looked at brain structure and function in patients with type I diabetes. It is known that acute hypoglycaemia has an acute detrimental effect on brain function,[38] although a recent study suggests that recurrent exposure to severe hypoglycaemia in young people with type I diabetes mellitus has no detrimental effects on brain structure or function.[39] Chronic hyperglycaemia (inferred by the presence of diabetic retinopathy), however, does appear to have an effect on brain structure and function, in that it is associated with small focal white matter changes in the basal ganglia and significant cognitive disadvantage.[39]

8.4   Oesophageal Complications

Oesophageal abnormalities in patients with diabetes are common, but what is clear from studies is that, despite the high prevalence of disorders of oesophageal motility in diabetes, there is not a clear increase in oesophageal symptoms. It is possible that this is due to a possible visceral afferent neuropathy in these patients.

Motor abnormalities

Oesophageal manometric and scintigraphic studies show that oesophageal transit is delayed in 40–60 per cent of diabetic patients, with a decrease in amplitude and number of peristaltic waves and an increase in simultaneous and non-propagated waves.[40] Rarely, marked abnormalities of motility, such as diffuse oesophageal spasm, are seen in diabetic patients. Additionally, lower oesophageal sphincter pressure is reduced compared with controls, suggesting a predisposition to gastro-oesophageal reflux.[41] It has been hypothesized that these effects are secondary to vagal neuropathy, since the vagus is the major efferent supply to the oesophagus. In support of this there is demyelination and loss of Schwann cells in the parasympathetic fibres of long standing type I diabetic patients.[42]

Sensory abnormalities

Decreased oesophageal sensory perception has been described in diabetic patients and may explain why, despite the high prevalence of motor dysfunction, this group remain relatively asymptomatic. Conversely, Rayner et al.[43] have demonstrated increased cortical evoked perception to low-pressure balloon distension in the oesophagus during acute hyperglycaemia, suggesting that under these conditions there is either increased peripheral perception or increased central processing. In essence, chronicity of diabetes may result in impairment of sensation, whilst acute hyperglycaemia enhances sensory awareness.

Gastro-oesophageal reflux

Perhaps unsurprisingly, given the prevalence of ineffective oesophageal peristalsis and decreased lower oesophageal pressure, gastro-oesophageal reflux (GORD) is more common in diabetic patients than matched controls. Even in asymptomatic patients, studies suggest that up to 40 per cent of diabetic patients have significant GORD,[44] although there is no evidence that the prevalence of oesophagitis is higher.

Dysphagia

Dysphagia describes the inability to swallow a solid or liquid bolus and is associated with a feeling of the bolus becoming 'stuck' before reaching the stomach. It is often described as being retrosternal, although localization by symptoms is notoriously imprecise. It is more common for dysphagia to be secondary to a mechanical obstruction such as peptic stricture or tumour than to be secondary to oesophageal dysmotility, and investigations should be tailored to rule out these organic causes before any functional studies are pursued. There is no evidence for an increase in oesophageal malignancy in diabetics *per se*, but there should be a low threshold for endoscopic investigation in the presence of dysphagia, especially in type II diabetics who are obese and more theoretically at risk of malignancy.

Candidal oesophagitis

This condition is not uncommon in diabetic patients and should be suspected in any diabetic patient who presents with painful swallowing (odynophagia). When severe it can present as dysphagia and in these circumstances prompt endoscopic evaluation is required. Endoscopic appearances are diagnostic with fluffy white exudates on the oesophageal mucosa. If there is doubt, brushings can be taken at the time of endoscopy, with microscopy revealing the fungal hyphae. Treatment with oral antifungals will often have a dramatic effect on symptoms and can be commenced empirically prior to endoscopy if there is any delay. Previously this condition was diagnosed frequently on double contrast barium swallow (which also gave a subjective view of motility), but endoscopy would now be the investigation of choice.

Psychological effects

The prevalence of anxiety and depression in diabetic patients with oesophageal contraction abnormailities (87 per cent) is significantly greater than in those without (21 per cent).[45] This suggests that there may be a psychiatric association with oesophageal motor abnormalities in at least some diabetic patients. It has been postulated that this may arise from abnormalities of arousal and secondary activation of autonomic outflow from the higher centres.

Investigations

Oesophageal symptoms include heartburn, acid regurgitation, odynophagia and dysphagia. In a diabetic population there will be a higher prevalence of GORD and in the setting of severe heartburn an early endoscopy is warranted to confirm the presence or absence of oesophagitis or Barrett's oesophagus (pre-malignant dysplastic change in the distal oesophagus related to chronic acid exposure). In the absence of inflammation or in the setting of continuing symptoms despite adequate acid suppression, oesophageal manometry and ambulatory 24 h pH studies should be considered. In addition to defining the amount of acid refluxed into the oesophagus, ambulatory pH studies reveal whether or not symptoms coincide with acid exposure, implying a significant relationship between observed acid exposure and symptoms. Odynophagia may be present in the absence of any mucosal inflammation, but its presence in a diabetic patient suggests possible candidiasis and the patient should be referred for endoscopy with empirical therapy if there is a delay. Dysphagia, as with non-diabetic patients, requires urgent investigation with endoscopy to rule out a mechanical cause. Some gastroenterologists will perform a contrast swallow prior to this to define the anatomy first. In the absence of mechanical blockage further investigations such as manometry or scintigraphy will define motility abnormalities. However, since these investigations are invasive and not widely available, it is reasonable to consider empirical therapy (see below) without testing.

Treatment

Symptoms of heartburn should be treated conventionally with acid suppression. Odynophagia secondary to candidiasis is treated with a one week course of an antifungal such as Nystatin 1–3 million units 6 hourly or fluconazole 100 mg daily. Treating motility disturbances is more problematic. There is limited evidence of efficacy of prokinetic medication on oesophageal symptoms in diabetics. Cisapride, a $5HT_4$ agonist which has now been withdrawn for the market due to its potential cardiotoxicity, has acute effects on oesophageal transit but does not appear to improve symptoms with chronic use.[46] Domperidone has been shown to increase oesophageal emptying in those with delayed transit, but has a variable effect on symptoms. There is also little evidence for the use of metoclopramide or erythromycin in this setting.

8.5 Stomach Complications

As previously alluded to, the effect of diabetes on gastric function has been the subject of study for many years, and until recently was thought to be a relatively rare problem. It is becoming increasingly evident that both hyperglycaemia *per se* as well as diabetes can have a profound effect on gastric function. Kassander, who initially named the syndrome 'gastroparesis diabeticorum', suggested that 'this syndrome . . . is more frequently overlooked than diagnosed', a view which is supported by recent studies.

There is evidence of delayed gastric emptying in 30–50 per cent of diabetic patients who have undergone gastric emptying studies.[47] This, however, does not mean that up to 50 per cent of diabetic patients have severe upper gut symptoms, and indeed there is poor correlation between symptoms and the presence of delayed gastric emptying.[48] However, symptoms of gastric dysfunction may result from abnormal accommodation in response to a meal, as much as to the delay in expulsion of that meal. This may be a physiological basis for this lack of correlation between symptoms and gastric emptying which spills over into the lack of an effective therapy for these symptoms.

At its worst diabetic gastroparesis can have a significant effect on quality of life and may lead to repeated hospital admissions. The abnormal gastric emptying results in variable absorption of glucose and hence major problems with glycaemic control. This can lead to a self perpetuating cycle of symptomatic gastroparesis and poor glycaemic control. Although a recent study demonstrates little change in degree of gastric emptying over time,[49] gastroparesis remains a very difficult problem to treat.

Gastric function

The stomach acts not only as a conduit for the digestion of food, but has a very specific regional function. On first swallowing food, the stomach first acts as a reservoir, with an initial receptive relaxation followed by a prolonged accommodation allowing the stomach to distend without significant increases in pressure. This accommodation is mostly related to gastric fundal relaxation. The food is then propagated by tonic contraction of the proximal stomach towards the pylorus. During this digestive phase, contraction waves arise from the pacemaker region in the greater curvature of the stomach at a rate of three per minute. Some, but not all, of these lead to contractions which sweep food down to the antrum, where strong contractions against a closed pylorus lead to grinding of the food particles. The passage of food particles to the duodenum is then dependent on antroduodenal and pyloric coordination. The pylorus will initially open slightly to allow the passage of liquid, and then particles of 1–2 mm. Wider opening and propulsion of larger indigestible particles occur in the interdigestive period. During the interdigestive period the stomach undergoes motor patterns which occur in a cyclical fashion and are termed the migrating motor complex. Phase I consists of motor quiescence and lasts around 40 min. This is followed by phase II for approximately 50 min, consisting of irregular contractions. Phase III, in which indigestible matter is propagated caudally from the distal stomach and proximal small intestine, is a brief complex of propagated waves at three cycles per minute, which originate primarily in the antrum.

The rate at which stomach emptying occurs in health is therefore dependent on many factors. As well as neuropathic damage to any of the neuronally controlled processes above, the type of nutrients ingested will affect gastric emptying. High-fat meals will slow gastric emptying through the enhanced release of factors such as cholecystokinin via vagally mediated chemoreceptors in the duodenum.

Pathophysiology

Patients with diabetic gastroparesis exhibit multiple motor and sensory abnormalities of the upper gut function: antral hypomotility, altered intragastric distribution of ingested food, abnormal intestinal contraction, increased fundic compliance and abnormal gastric sensation. These abnormalities have been demonstrated in patients following vagotomy and it was assumed for some time that 'autovagotomy' accounted for the majority of problems encountered. Vagal integrity is necessary for migrating motor complex (MMC) origination in the stomach and the absence of antral MMCs in symptomatic diabetic gastroparetic patients supports this further.[50] Additionally, enteric neuropathy and abnormalities in interstitial cells of Cajal have been described in this condition (see Section 8.1), and may contribute to the aetiopathogenesis. A recent report has suggested that there may be an associated auto-immune state in diabetic patients with gastroparesis, with the observation of autoantibodies to calcium channel receptors in gastric smooth muscle cells.[51]

Hyperglycaemia has a profound effect on gut function and has been found to slow gastric emptying (Figure 8.1), reduce post-prandial antral contractions[52] and alter proximal stomach perception.[53] Furthermore, hyperglycaemia may affect the efficacy of therapy through attenuation of the effect of erythromycin.[54] There is also evidence to suggest that hyperglycaemia has an effect on vagal function. Following a meal, there is an increase in the plasma levels of pancreatic polypeptide increase (a marker of intra-abdominal vagal function). This response is attenuated in hyperglycaemia, suggesting reversible vagal efferent dysfunction.[55]

Diagnosis

The diagnosis of diabetic gastroparesis requires an objective demonstration of delayed gastric emptying, as symptom correlation is poor. In a recent study, the

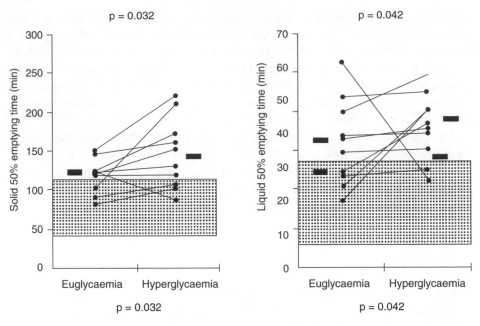

Figure 8.1 Graphs representing the delay during hyperglycaemia in solid and liquid gastric emptying in patients with type I diabetes mellitus. Reproduced from Fraser *et al.*, *Diabetologia*, 1990; 33, 678, with permission of Springer-Verlag

only symptom that correlated with the presence of delayed gastric emptying was bloating, but not nausea or vomiting.[47]

The 'gold-standard' test for gastric emptying is radio-isotope scintigraphy, although the development of other techniques may soon supercede this. Scintigraphic measurement was initially inaccurate between centres as the technique was not standardized, a problem that has now been resolved. The radiation exposure is not excessive, being comparable to an abdominal radiograph. Alternative means of studying gastric function include MRI, ultrasound and the use of carbon breath tests. The latter is non-invasive and may present a useful office-based technique.[56] Radio-opaque marker ingestion followed by abdominal X-ray is a technique that has been used but is not accurate and gives no differentiation between solid and liquid phase emptying.

As well as investigating gastric emptying, we can also investigate other motor and sensory abnormalities. The use of the barostat to give us accurate volume and pressure distensions allows testing of sensation throughout the stomach, and ultrasound techniques (as well as the barostat) allow a closer assessment of gastric accommodation. Abnormalities in electrical conduction within the stomach wall can be investigated by electrogastrography, which will demonstrate any tachy- or bradyarrhythmias affecting the gastric slow waves. Such elctrophysiological abnormalities have been demonstrated in gastroparesis.

However, the routine use of all of these investigations in diabetic patients who present with upper GI symptoms cannot be recommended in the first instance. In subjects presenting with recurrent vomiting, an upper GI endoscopy should be performed to rule out mechanical obstruction. Electrolyte imbalance, thyroid and adrenal dysfunction can all exacerbate symptoms and these should be checked. As mentioned above, it is vital that blood sugar control is as tight as possible, and this should be discussed with the patient. It is only after these investigations have been completed that an objective measurement of gastric emptying becomes necessary (Figure 8.2).

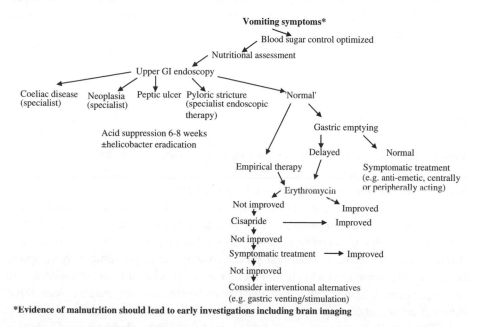

Figure 8.2 Flow chart of the initial evaluation of the diabetic patient presenting with vomiting. Note that malnutrition and weight loss should lead to prompt investigation, including brain imaging if all other investigations are normal

Treatment

Diabetic gastroparesis presents a major management problem. The primary goal should be to improve symptoms, since an improvement in symptoms does not always correlate with improved gastric emptying. Improvement in gastric emptying would be an advantage to allow a predictable and physiological delivery of nutrients to the small bowel, and hence more predictable and stable post-prandial blood glucose concentrations and insulin requirements. To date, however, we have no therapy that predictably addresses both these goals. In conjunction with pharmacological therapy, it is vitally important that nutrition is maintained. Although there are no studies confirming the efficacy of dietary manipulation, it is intuitive that foods that slow gastric emptying will worsen gastroparesis in symptomatic periods. A low-fibre, low-fat liquid diet taken in small amounts frequently is the least likely to aggravate symptoms and should be tried initially. If this cannot be tolerated and the patient is malnourished, nutrition may have to be by jejunal tube feeding, bypassing the stomach. This can be placed endoscopically or fluoroscopically and should be considered only after a successful trial of nasoenteric feeding, since there is a high prevalence of small intestinal motility in these patients. Parenteral feeding should be used only as a last resort, since there are attendant major risks associated with central feeding, especially line sepsis There are clearly problems associated with blood glucose control when feeds are administered overnight (as is customary in non-diabetic subjects), and it may be easier at first to administer the feeds over a 24 h period to get a better idea of insulin requirements.

Prokinetic medication

Prokinetic medications are the current mainstay of therapy for gastroparesis. These drugs target a variety of receptors to increase gastric emptying. The best investigated agents are metoclopramide and cisapride ($5HT_4$ receptor agonists), metoclopramide and domperidone (dopamine-2 antagonists), and more recently erythromycin (a motilin analogue). In one formal meta-analysis of the use of currently available prokinetics in gastroparesis, Sturm et al.[57] found that in double-blind, controlled studies, cisapride produced a mean improvement in symptom score of only 8 per cent, whereas metoclopramide produced a mean improvement of 36 per cent. It should be noted that these figures are comparable with those attained by placebo.

Unfortunately, none of these drugs appear to have long-term efficacy in alleviating symptoms, and at best only a variable effect on gastric emptying. Some of their effect may be on other gastric functions such as fundic relaxation. It has been proposed, for example, that one of the reasons motilin analogues may not be as effective as expected is that they lead to fundic contraction. The studies into the efficacy of these medications vary in treatment duration and end point, and blood sugar control has not usually been accounted for.

Motilin is a peptide hormone produced in the upper GI tract. It enhances gastric and upper gut motility, and it is hoped that production of motilin analogues will improve treatment of conditions that involve upper gut motor dysfunction, including diabetic gastroparesis. Erythromycin increases antral motility and does so by its action at the motilin receptor.[58] It has been shown to improve gastric emptying in gastroparesis.[59] However, it is an antibiotic and the search has been on for effective derivative compounds which are as effective but lack antibiotic properties. Several have been shown to be effective pre-clinically,[60–62] but have not been demonstrated to have a long-term effect on symptoms. This may be due to tachyphylaxis of drugs which have a relatively long half-life or indeed because motilin analogues have some detrimental effects on symptoms themselves (via fundic contraction). To date the efficacy of this class of drug has proved disappointing, but studies with new agents continue.

Despite the poor efficacy over time, the use of prokinetics in symptomatic patients should be considered in patients who remain symptomatic despite dietary modification. Cisapride is now available only on a named-patient basis in the UK. A trial of this or another of the prokinetics is worthwhile, to be continued only if the patient has symptomatic relief. In the acute setting of a hospital admission, erythromycin intravenously starting at doses of 500 mg b.d. or t.d.s. should be considered to abort an attack. This can then be weaned to low doses (e.g. 125 mg b.d.) in the long-term, with there being some evidence for greater efficacy with the drug in suspension form.[63]

Gastric neurostimulation

Gastric neurostimulation involves the subcutaneous implantation of a device at either laparotomy or laparoscopy. The device is approximately the size of a cardiac pacemaker, comprising an impulse generator connected to two electrodes. The electrodes are placed deep into the muscularis propria 1 cm apart about 9.5–10.5 cm from the pylorus along the greater curvature of the stomach (Enterra[TM] Medtronic, Minneapolis, MN, USA). During the procedure, an intra-operative endoscopy confirms the wires have not been put in too far and breached the gastric mucosa. The electrical stimulation is set at a higher frequency than the normal gastric pacemaker slow waves (12 vs three cycles per minute), and utilizes low energy levels (300 ms pulse width, 4–5 mA). An initial report suggests that this therapy leads to a greater than 50 per cent decrease in nausea and vomiting in three-quarters of subjects (Figure 8.3). The device is now approved by the FDA in the USA for use in gastroparetic patients refractory to medical therapy. However, the mechanism of action of the stimulator remains unclear, as there is a poor correlation between gastric emptying and symptom improvement. This again raises the possibility of some action at an enteric or afferent nerve level, although studies are ongoing to elucidate the mechanism.[64]

Surgery

In some patients with intractable symptoms, gastrectomy is a treatment option, usually with resection of most of the stomach with a Roux-en-Y loop. The procedure is associated with significant morbidity and should be thought of as

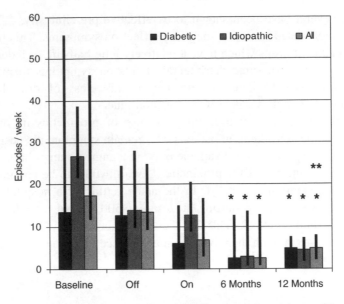

Figure 8.3 Graph illustrating the weekly vomiting frequency for patients with gastroparesis before and during gastric stimulation when the stimulator was on or off (double-blind period), and also at 6 and 12 months during the open phase when the stimulator remained on. There was a significant decrease in vomiting frequency for all types of gastroparesis at 6 and 12 months follow-up (*$p < 0.05$ vs baseline). Reproduced from Abell *et al.*, *Gastroenterology* 2003; **125**: 426 with kind permission from Elsevier Science

a last resort when all medical therapies have failed. Careful patient selection is the key, and in a small number of refractory cases the procedure can be beneficial.[65]

Other therapies

A sub-group of gastroparetic patients have pylorospasm that will affect gastric emptying, which can be demonstrated manometrically. It has been suggested that injection with 100–200 units of botulinum toxin A in four quadrants around the pylorus under endoscopic guidance is effective at relieving symptoms.[66] However, further studies are needed to define which patients will benefit from this therapy since it is expensive and the effect is only temporary and needs to be repeated. An alternative approach to pylorospasm is to consider balloon dilatation of the pylorus, although again the procedure is of limited efficacy and duration.[67]

The development of novel pharmacological therapies may prove beneficial in the future. The use of more specific $5HT_4$ agonists may improve the modest results seen with current prokinetics. In addition, novel motilin analogues show early promise.[60] Ghrelin, a neuropeptide secreted from the stomach, has been shown to increase stomach contractility in animal models, and may form a putative target for future drug innovation.[68,69]

8.6 Small Intestine

Abnormalities in small intestinal motility have been found to be present in up to 80 per cent of patients with long-standing diabetes.[31] The commonest abnormality is small intestinal transit delay in 23 per cent of patients in the largest series to date.[70] These abnormalities include a lack of MMCs commencing in the antrum, prolonged phasic non-propagated contractions, a decrease in the frequency and amplitude of duodenal and jejunal contractions and the failure of the small intestine to adopt a 'fed motility pattern' following meal ingestion. There is, however, poor correlation between these manometric findings and symptoms.

As with gastroparesis, these physiological abnormalities significantly alter the degree to which food is processed and absorbed. Glycaemic control can be improved by decreasing the post-prandial blood glucose peak, and addition of fibre to the diet has been shown to improve this in both type I and type II diabetes.[71,72] The effect of dietary fibre is to slow both gastric emptying and subsequent intestinal glucose absorption due to the increased intraluminal viscosity. Hyperglycaemia may have an effect on small intestinal sensory and motor physiology. In the small intestine, hyperglycaemia leads to a decrease in the number and propagation of pressure waves in the proximal small intestine,[73] and an increase in the perception of both chemical and mechanical luminal stimuli.[74]

Small bowel bacterial overgrowth

The normal proximal small bowel contains less than 10^5 bacteria per millilitre, with concentrations rising to around 10^8 in the distal small intestine. In situations where there is prolonged proximal small intestinal transit, either due to mechanical or dysmotility reasons, there can be an increase in bacteria to levels comparable with those found in the healthy colon, and this is termed small bowel bacterial overgrowth (SBBO).

In the healthy gut, bacterial levels are controlled in the proximal small bowel by gastric acid secretion and intestinal motility, of which the MMC ('the intestinal housekeeper') plays an important part. In diabetes, proximal small bowel dysmotility can lead to stagnation and increased colonisation. There may be a contributing role of immune abnormality, since patients with SBBO may have altered levels of secretory immunoglobulin A, and diabetes is associated with an immune paresis.

Bacterial overgrowth can lead to symptoms and malabsorption through a number of different mechanisms. Malabsorption of both macronutrients (fats and carbohydrates) as well as micronutrients (fat soluble vitamins and vitamin B_{12}) can occur. In addition, symptoms of increased gas and bloating may occur secondary to small intestinal fermentation.

In SBBO, bacteria in the proximal small intestine can deconjugate the bile salts that are needed for fat processing and furthermore the bacteria produce free bile acids which are readily absorbed. These bacterial-induced metabolic changes can lead to steatorrhoea, as well as possibly causing direct damage to the small bowel mucosa by the free bile acids themselves. This damage further limits the ability to the proximal small bowel to absorb nutrients. Fat-soluble vitamins A, D, E and K can be malabsorbed. With severe deficiencies, all of these can lead to clinical syndromes. Vitamin A deficiency can lead to night blindness, vitamin D deficiency to osteomalacia and vitamin K deficiency to a coagulopathy. All of these deficiencies are correctable.

Carbohydrate absorption may also be affected. Intraluminal digestion of carbohydrate by bacteria can exacerbate damage to the mucosa and decrease disaccharidase activity, further exacerbating malabsorption syndromes. In addition to the free bile acids described above, malabsorbed carbohydrate can then exacerbate symptoms as it is broken down in the colon to produce other organic acids and stimulate a secretory and osmotic diarrhoea.

Weight loss may occur secondary to both malabsorption and also the utilization of nutrients by bacteria. Some bacterial strains also utilize vitamin B_{12} and patients with SBBO are often vitamin B_{12}-deficient with the attendant neurological and haematological consequences. The B_{12} deficiency is offset to some extent by intrinsic bacterial production of the vitamin.

Diagnosis

SBBO should be considered in diabetic patients who have troublesome gastro-intestinal symptoms, especially if there is any clinical evidence of malabsorption. The 'gold standard' diagnostic test is jejunal aspiration and culture, since this allows the sensitivities of the organisms to be ascertained. However, this is an invasive procedure, and hence most units use a breath test as a surrogate marker for SBBO. Both the ^{14}C-cholylglycine and the ^{14}C-xylose breath test work by recording radiolabelled breath carbon dioxide in response to ingestion of a test meal containing either radiolabelled cholylglycine or xylose respectively. The former test used to be popular, but has a 30–40 per cent false negative rate and is less used now. The ^{14}C-xylose breath test has up to a 95 per cent sensitivity and 100 per cent specificity. The bacteria in the proximal small intestine break down the xylose and cause an early peak of radiolabelled carbon dioxide production, and any undigested xylose is absorbed, avoiding any subsequent fermentation in the colon, thus enhancing specificity.

As both of these breath tests use radiation, some units have adopted a hydrogen breath test. This test involves the ingestion of either lactulose or glucose and the recording of breath hydrogen which has been liberated by bacterial breakdown. Lactulose will normally lead to hydrogen production when it reaches the colon and hence this type of breath test shows a 'double peak' if bacteria are present in the small intestine, with the abnormal peak in breath hydrogen followed by the expected colonic peak. However, a significant proportion of the SBBO population (up to 40 per cent) carry bacteria that do not break down lactulose, resulting in a false negative result. This does not occur when using glucose, although the rapid absorption of glucose in the upper GI tract may bypass bacterial digestion and again lead to a false negative. The resting levels of breath hydrogen are also raised at baseline in up to 30 per cent of patients, making interpretation impossible.[75] The test results are affected by the ingestion of high-carbohydrate meals in the period before the test, and antibiotics and laxatives must be withheld. The hydrogen breath test does have the advantage of being a safe and non-invasive test avoiding exposure to radiation, but its low specificity and sensitivity make it unreliable.

Treatment

In order to treat SBBO effectively, the primary cause for gut stasis and overgrowth should be treated. Improving glycaemic control can improve upper gut dysmotility, but is unlikely to reverse all the abnormalities seen in diabetic patients. The mainstay of treatment remains antibiotics. The choice and regime of antibiotic needs to cover both anaerobic and aerobic bacteria and should be given in short or cyclical courses. Tetracycline has been used historically, but there is evidence of bacterial resistance and it is no longer an ideal first-line choice. An initial course of 10 days of amoxycillin–clavulinic acid, ciprofloxacin or doxycycline has been shown to be effective. In subjects with recurrent symptoms, these antibiotics can be used consecutively in a cyclical manner to avoid resistance.[75]

Probiotic therapy of SBBO is appealing for its safety profile and lack of risk of development of resistance. However, to date it has proved disappointing in this condition.[76] Attempts to clear the bacteria by using a prokinetic have been successful with cisapride in a small study,[77] but there is at this time little other data to suggest their use as first-line therapy.

Coeliac disease

As well as the effect of diabetes itself on the small intestine, adult patients with type I diabetes have a six times greater prevalence of coeliac disease, and in children with type I diabetes this prevalence is 15 times greater, suggesting a genetic linkage between these conditions. Shanahan *et al.*[70] showed that, in patients with type I diabetes and coeliac disease, HLA markers B8 and DR3 were common, with their presence conferring more risk of developing both diseases. Coeliac disease is the most common small bowel enteropathy in the Western world and classically presents with diarrhoea and weight loss and anaemia. The anaemia can be caused by malabsorption of iron, folic acid or vitamin B_{12}, and all of these levels should be monitored and supplemented as required. However, up to 30 per cent of subjects can be asymptomatic. Taken together with the prevalence data, this is persuasive evidence that there should be a low threshold for investigation of coeliac diasease in diabetic patients.

The gold standard investigation for coeliac disease is small bowel biopsies from the duodenum or jejunum which show the pathognomic features of subtotal villous atrophy and an increase in epithelial lymphocytes. Anti-endomysial antibodies (EMA) are over 85 per cent sensitive and up to 100 per cent specific and can be used as a screening tool.[79] However, some patients with coeliac disease have a selective IgA deficiency, which may be important since most laboratories will test for the IgA EMA. Therefore if there is a strong suspicion then the IgA levels should themselves be checked and possibly an IgG as well. Recently the antigen recognized by EMA, tissue transglutaminase, has been discovered and the use of human recombinant transglutaminase antigen has been proved to be more sensitive (91%) and just as specific as the EMA test.[79] For now, though, EMA remains the initial antibody test of choice, although this may change.

Treatment of coeliac disease is the life-long exclusion of wheat, rye, barley and prolamins from the diet under the supervision of a dietician. With this regime most patients normalize the changes seen in the small bowel mucosa. A small proportion of patients do not respond to a strictly adhered to exclusion diet, and there is persisting histological evidence of disease. These patients are candidates for immunosuppressive therapy, initially with steroids (with the stipulation of careful glucose monitoring in diabetic patients), and possibly azathioprine in the tiny minority who need long-term treatment.

8.7 Colon

The most frequently reported GI symptom in diabetics is constipation.[80] Under normal circumstances, the function of the colon is to receive and ferment undigested food and to absorb back fluid and some nutrients. This results in the rectum being presented with predominantly indigestible material and bacteria. Contents are mixed and churned throughout the colon with primarily non-propagated contractions. Peristaltic contractions move the stool slowly in a caudal direction, and from time to time giant peristaltic movements or 'high-amplitude propagated contractions' cause mass movement of stool. These occur during defaecation, but are often also initiated on waking or at times of eating (the 'gastro-colic reflex'). In a group of diabetic patients with constipation, this gastro-colic reflex was found to be decreased or absent. Administration of neostigmine (an anticholinesterase inhibitor, which increases the concentration of available acetylcholine), results in a similar colonic contractile response in diabetic patients as controls. Since the muscle function appeared normal, the suggestion is that the abnormality is at an enteric or autonomic nerve level.[32] Abnormalities of the enteric nervous system and of interstitial cells of Cajal have been described in patients with slow-transit constipation, but not specifically in patients with diabetes.

Diagnosis

The diagnosis of constipation is made by symptom criteria and, for the purposes of consensus, the Rome II criteria were formulated. A full history and examination should be performed, including digital rectal examination. If the onset of constipation is abrupt or associated with rectal bleeding, then a mechanical cause should be ruled out with colonic imaging (preferably colonoscopy). It can also be of value to establish whether there is an objective measure of slow whole-gut transit which can be assessed with a transit study. This is a simple investigation, entailing ingestion of three sets of radio-opaque markers over 3 days followed by an abdominal radiograph on the fifth day to assess how many markers remain. In addition, blood tests should be sent to exclude any metabolic changes which can be associated with constipation such as hypothyroidism and hypercalcaemia. Anorectal physiology can be contributory, since it allows testing of the recto-anal inhibitory reflex (RAIR) in those with long-standing constipation. The presence of the RAIR excludes a diagnosis of Hirschsprung's disease.

Generally, in a young diabetic patient with mild symptoms of constipation it is acceptable to advise lifestyle changes (regular meals, increase fluid intake togreater than 2 l per day) and an increase in fibre intake, and only if that fails is a trial of a laxative appropriate (see below), prior to further exhaustative investigation.

Treatment

Other than advising tight blood sugar control, treatment of constipation remains symptomatic as for non-diabetics patients. Initially lifestyle advice can be helpful, including an increase in dietary fibre in the diet and taking adequate oral fluid each day. The use of laxatives can then be in the form of an osmotic agent (especially if transit is slow) or stimulant laxatives for occasional on-demand use. There is no evidence supporting the use of one type of laxative over another, but a trial of monotherapy with one agent should be considered, with an emphasis on the avoidance of polypharmacy. There is little evidence in the literature to support the long-term efficacy of laxative medication in the diabetic population, although chronic use is not associated with significant adverse effects in the overwhelming majority of constipated patients. There is also no good evidence to support the use of prokinetic medication, or newer drugs such as the $5HT_4$ agonist, tegaserod in patients with diabetes. The most effective therapy for refractory cases is biofeedback. Behavioural therapy (biofeedback) is effective in around two-thirds of patients with constipation that has not improved with lifestyle changes or laxatives. The classical methodology involves operant conditioning with patients given either audio or visual feedback of muscle activity during attempted evacuation and relaxation of the anorectum. Patients are also instructed on how to employ relaxation techniques and use the diaphragm and abdominal muscles appropriately to facilitate defaecation.

8.8   Anorectal Function

Anorectal dysfunction is more common in diabetic patients with evidence of autonomic neuropathy. However, it should be remembered that symptoms of anorectal dysfunction (faecal urgency and incontinence) may result from diarrhoea and transit acceleration related to non-neuropathic diabetic factors. Thus, anorectal symptoms may occur in diabetic patients with only a short duration of disease.

Diagnosis

Urgency and faecal incontinence are troublesome and miserable symptoms that are often missed as they are not asked for directly and patients are embarrassed to bring them up in the consultation. Symptoms of faecal urgency can be exacerbated by diarrhoea and a thorough history should be sought to see if this is the case. In addition, the anorectal area should be assessed physiologically and structurally. Digital examination is only of limited value in this. Endoanal ultrasound allows assessment of the external and internal sphincters and will reveal any defects or degeneration of the muscle. However, even with some marked structural abnormalities function can be preserved, and this can be quantified with anorectal physiological testing. Assessment of normal subjects during hyperglycaemia has demonstrated inhibition of internal and external anal sphincter function and heightened rectal sensitivity. In a diabetic population impaired external and internal anal sphincter function has been demonstrated in association with rectal hyposensation in one study.[81] Additionally, acute hyperglycaemia inhibits external anal sphincter function and decreases rectal compliance.[82] Hence diabetes itself and acute hyperglycaemia can increase the chance of faecal incontinence. The fact that symptoms are improved by biofeedback suggests that this is not a permanent neuropathic phenomenon.

Treatment

Treatment of episodes of urgency and incontinence should look at dealing with the underlying cause. There is good evidence that good glycaemic control will be helpful. If the predominant problem is diarrhoea then investigation and treatment of this may alleviate symptoms. Symptomatic treatment with loperamide or similar drug is helpful and decreases symptoms of urgency. Used judiciously, this is effective and safe. Biofeedback has been specifically shown to be a successful therapy in this patient group.[81]

8.9 Pancreatic

The pancreas obviously has a central role in the pathophysiology of diabetes. Hence it is no surprise that other pancreatic diseases can lead to a diabetic state, in particular acute and chronic pancreatitis. The former probably initially via increased levels of glucagon and epinephrine rather than a decrease in insulin production. In the chronic situation, chronic fibrosis of the whole organ leads to islet cell damage and a decrease in insulin production.

During episodes of acute pancreatitis, amylase levels are markedly raised. This can be attenuated in long-term diabetic patients who have a lower amylase output, but conversely, the diabetic ketoacidotic patient with a high serum amylase should not be assumed to have pancreatitis. Hyperamylasaemia occurs in the setting of ketoacidosis in the absence of any pancreatic inflammation and this should be remembered when assessing the ketoacidotic patient with abdominal pain. The initial management should always involve treatment of the acidosis.

As well as endocrine dysfunction (predominantly in type I diabetes, but to some extent in type II), there is a surprisingly high prevalence of pancreatic exocrine dysfunction in diabetic subjects. Pancreatic exocrine insufficiency is found in 65–80 per cent of diabetic patients. Despite this, symptomatic exocrine insufficiency is actually quite rare, since there is a large reserve built into the system. However, episodic steathorrhoea, especially with high-fat meals, may occur.

The reason for exocrine insufficiency in diabetes is probably multifactorial. Hyperglycaemia itself has an inhibitory effect on exocrine function in normal subjects. The lack of insulin as a trophic factor in type I diabetes is probably contributory and finally microangiopathy and fibrosis surrounding the islet cells will affect the exocrine cells.

Pancreatic carcinoma is thought to occur more frequently in diabetics with the pooled relative risk in a meta-analysis being 2.1 when compared with non-diabetics.[83] The presence of pancreatic cancer can also lead to an insulin-resistant diabetic state which resolves with tumour resection.

Diagnosis

Pancreatic exocrine insufficiency should be suspected when steatorrhoea is reported and this should be confirmed by performing a 3 day faecal collection to look for both mass (diarrhoea is confirmed if daily stool weight is greater than 200 g) and fat to confirm fat malabsorption (greater than 3 g fat per day on normal diet). The gold standard tests for exocrine insufficiency involve duodenal intubation and are therefore invasive. A faecal elastase-1 is a marker of insufficiency and can be used in support of the faecal fat findings. In a chronic pancreatitis population, faecal elastase-1 has been shown to have a sensitivity ranging from 0–65 per cent in mild disease to 33–100 per cent in severe disease with a specificity of 29–95 per cent.[84] In a recent study, 36 per cent of asymptomatic diabetic patients were found to have low faecal elastase-1 levels compared with 5 per cent of healthy controls.[85] There are other direct and indirect non-invasive tests of exocrine insufficiency. In addition to faecal elastase-1, non-invasive direct tests include a serum trypsin assay and faecal chymotrypsin. Indirect tests include the pancreolauryl test, the bentiromide test, quantitative faecal fat excretion and faecal fat analysis. The average sensitivity, however, for all of these non-invasive tests outside the setting of severe chronic pancreatitis is 50 per cent,[85,86] limiting their use as screening tools. The pancreas should be imaged for evidence of chronic damage with an ultrasound and, if a tumour suspected, imaged by CT as well.

Treatment

Replacement of pancreatic enzymes should begin with between 25 000 and 40 000 units of lipase with each meal using pH-sensitive pancreatin microspheres. There may be some benefit of the addition of a proton pump inhibitor or an H2 antagonist to help prevent gastric digestion of the enzymes.[87,88] The dose of pancreatic enzyme supplementation can then be titrated up until malabsorption improves, with a close eye kept on glycaemic control, since better nutrient handling will clearly affect this.

8.10   Hepatobiliary

Liver in diabetes

Glycogenic infiltration

In poorly controlled type I diabetic patients hepatomegaly is present in up to 60 per cent of individuals secondary to glycogen infiltration. This is reversible and will respond to appropriate insulin therapy to maintain tight blood sugar control.

Diagnosis is by liver biopsy, but this can be avoided if appropriate therapy resolves the hepatomegaly and an ultrasound has previously been performed to rule out any intrahepatic lesions.

Non-alcoholic fatty liver disease

Non-alcoholic fatty liver disorder encompasses a spectrum of liver disease ranging from hepatic steatosis to steatohepatitis and even cirrhosis. It is a highly prevalent condition throughout the Western world, with an estimated prevalence of up to 23 per cent in the USA.[89]

By definition non-alcoholic fatty liver disease can only be diagnosed in the absence of a history of alcohol consumption, and this should be carefully sought. Fatty liver in the absence of inflammation is thought of as a benign condition which does not progress to chronic liver disease. However, in the presence of inflammation, the condition is known as non-alcoholic steatohepatitis (NASH), which can lead to cirrhosis. It is thought that between 10 and 40 per cent of NASH patients progress to chronic liver disease.[89]

The pathophysiology of this condition is not fully understood. Although it can occur in type I diabetic patients, NASH is predominantly a problem in type II obese diabetic patients. Insulin blocks mitochondrial fatty acid oxidation and this results in increased intracellular fatty acid deposition, a process which is increased in the hyperinsulinaemic insulin-resistant type II diabetic patient. Insulin resistance and disordered fatty acid metabolism are therefore likely to play a central role in this condition. What then initiates subsequent inflammation, necrosis and fibrosis is not clear, but abnormal cytokine production and oxidative stress leading to lipid peroxidation have been causally implicated.

Diagnosis of a fatty liver is initially made on imaging. Ultrasound is 80 per cent sensitive and 100 per cent specific for the bright liver associated with fatty change. CT scan without contrast shows increased attenuation of the liver when compared with the spleen.[90] However, imaging gives no information on whether inflammation is present and for this a liver biopsy is required. Eighty per cent of patients with NASH will have abnormal liver enzymes and, in the setting of a diabetic patient with abnormal liver enzymes, no history of alcohol use and no other evident cause for an inflammatory liver picture, a liver biopsy is advised to document the degree of inflammation and fibrosis.

The essential first step in the treatment of NASH is to tighten control of any associated conditions, specifically diabetes and hyperlipidaemia. Gradual weight loss will help, but should not be done quickly since this can aggravate the condition and in rare cases has precipitated hepatic failure.

A number of drug therapy strategies have been considered in treating this common problem. Drugs aimed at decreasing triglyceride levels and cholesterol levels have studied due to their success in animal models. However, a 12 month trial of clofibrate failed to show any improvement in liver enzymes and liver histology in 16 patients with NASH.[91] Atorvastatin has been demonstrated to be effective in improving both of these parameters, but only in a small open-label study.[92]

Reduction of insulin resistance has been attempted using either a biguanide (metformin) or the newer thiazolidinediones. Metformin has been used as it sensitizes peripheral target tissues to insulin and decreases hepatic glucose production. In the small studies done to date, however, no improvement in liver histology has been observed.[93] Thiazolidinediones have direct insulin sensitizing effects and it was hoped that these would be more effective.[94] Unfortunately, the initial drug (troglitazone) had to be withdrawn after over 60 hepatic failure-related deaths. Newer drugs in this class such as rosiglitazone and piaglitazone do show promise, but further studies are needed to confirm their effectiveness and safety profile. For the time being, routine use of these drugs in NASH cannot be advised outside a trial setting.

Treatment with cytoprotective drugs such as vitamin E and ursodeoxycholic acid have also proved disappointing. A recent double-blind randomized controlled trial of the latter failed to show any change in liver enzymes or liver histology.[95]

At this time, therefore, treatment options remain limited. Diabetic patients should be advised with regard to weight loss and low-lipid diets, and as with other complications advised to keep as good a glycaemic control as possible. The cumulative incidence of chronic non-alcoholic liver disease is significantly higher in patients with diabetes[96] (Figure 8.4).

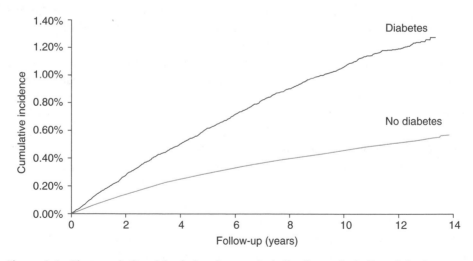

Figure 8.4 The cumulative risk of chronic non-alcoholic disease including cirrhosis among veteran patients hospitalized between 1985 and 1990 and a follow-up period that ended in 2002. Chronic non-alcoholic liver disease was significantly higher in patients with diabetes ($p < 0.0001$). Reproduced from El-Serag *et al.*, *Gastroenterology* 2004; **126**: 463 with kind permission from Elsevier

Other liver disorders

There is a slight increase in the prevalence of autoimmune hepatitis in the diabetic population, and in the work-up of a diabetic patient with abnormal liver biochemistry auto-antibodies including anti-mitochondrial (for primary biliary cirrhosis) and anti-smooth muscle antibodies should be sent.

Hepatitis B and C are also more prevalent in the diabetic population, possibly due to greater possible parenteral drug and blood product exposure, and appropriate viral antigens and antibodies should be checked for. This is important, as even in the absence of hepatitis B or C, a recent study has demonstrated a hazard rate ratio of 2.16 of hepatocellular carcinoma in men with diabetes when compared with controls.[96]

Haemochromatosis can lead to the onset of diabetes secondary to deposition of iron in the pancreas and liver. The combination of this and skin deposition led to the classical description of 'diabete bronzé'. Diagnosis is initially on blood testing with a transferrin saturation of greater than 50 per cent (and a raised ferritin). The gold standard, however, is liver biopsy with measurement of the dry liver weight of iron. It is now also possible to test for the most common mutations of the *HFE* gene.

Liver disease causing hyper- and hypoglycaemia

Cirrhotic liver disease can be associated with problems of both hyper- and hypoglycaemia. The former is commonly seen following a meal and may reflect in part peripheral insulin resistance and disordered glycogen production. Hypoglycaemia is often a problem in encephalopathic states, when decreased energy intake, impaired insulin breakdown and impaired glucose production are probably all involved.

8.11   Biliary Disorders

For many years it was felt that there was a higher prevalence of gallstones in diabetic patients than in normal controls. Historically, in fact, some clinicians advised prophylactic cholecystectomy in all diabetic patients since they appeared to do worse following surgery for acute cholecystitis.[97] However, it appears that much of the increased mortality was due to peri-operative care rather than diabetes *per se*, and this is certainly no longer advised.

The difficulty in judging whether gallstones are more prevalent in diabetic populations is predominantly because obesity is a risk factor for gallstone formation and much of the increased prevalence of gallstones is explained by the prevalence of obesity in the type 2 diabetes cohort. Once this co-factor is accounted for in statistical analysis, the relative risk of gallstones is similar in diabetic and non-diabetic subjects.

Gall bladder motility is affected in some diabetic patients, especially those with autonomic neuropathy.[98,99] Gall bladder emptying is also delayed in hyperglycaemia.[100] These motility factors do not seem to be clinically significant and there is no evidence that the prevalence of gallstones is secondary to chronic glycaemic control.

In summary, asymptomatic gallstones in a diabetic patient do not warrant prophylactic cholecystectomy. Acute cholecystitis should be treated as per a non-diabetic individual, but early surgery is suggested for the diabetic patient. Gallstone biliary obstruction should be managed by endoscopic retrograde cholepancreatography with stone clearance and/or stenting as would be the case for the non-diabetic patient.

8.12   Diabetic Diarrhoea

The aetiology of diarrhoea in the diabetic population can be multifactorial and the assessment of the patient should therefore take this into account (Figure 8.5). It is

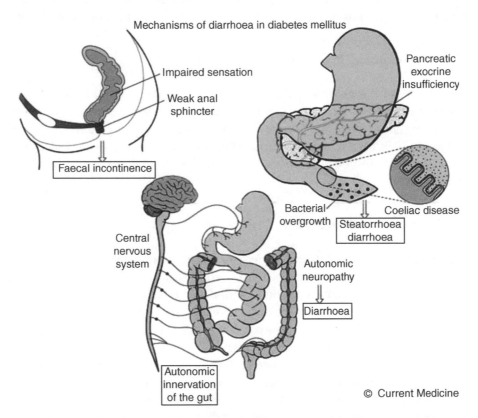

Figure 8.5   The presentation of diarrhoea in the diabetic patient is often multifactorial, and this should be addressed in the initial evaluation of symptoms. Reproduced from *Feldman's GastroAtlas* online, Figure 4.30. Vol. 7, (2004), with permission of Current Medicine Inc., Philadelphia

not clear whether the prevalence is higher in type 1 or 2 diabetic patients. Metformin use can often precipitate loose stool and the onset of symptoms in relation to starting this drug as well as others that can lead to diarrhoea should always be ascertained. When assessing any patient with diarrhoea it is first important to take a full history and establish the chronology, frequency and volume of diarrhoea. Diarrhoea is defined as a stool output of greater than 200 g per day, but many people will feel they have diarrhoea when they are passing loose stools or even small amounts of stool frequently. This is important since the aetiology of symptoms will be completely different. For example, we know that anorectal function can be affected in diabetic patients, and this may present as a constant feeling of urgency and multiple trips to the toilet. Equally diabetic patients are as likely as the general population to have irritable bowel syndrome, a functional disorder often associated with symptoms of rectal dissatisfaction (sensation of incomplete emptying, urgency and increased stool frequency).

As well as a precise history of the type of symptoms experienced, the chronicity should be established, as this may indicate whether there is a need to exclude an organic colonic cause for the diarrhoea. The history should also identify whether there is a nocturnal component, whether the diarrhoea is associated with incontinence, and whether there has been any foreign travel or ingestion of potentially spoiled food prior to its onset. It should be remembered that, despite the many abnormalities described in the gut, the most common causes of diarrhoea remain infective. The stool should therefore always be sent for culture and microscopy and in the population that have taken recent antibiotic therapy, the stool should be analysed for *Clostridium difficile* toxin.

Other causes of diarrhoea in the diabetic patient include disordered autonomically mediated intestinal secretion and motility. This can result in increased contractions and hence diarrhoea. Alternatively motility may be reduced, predisposing to small bowel bacterial overgrowth and possible bile salt malabsorption and hence causing diarrhoea. Autoimmune diseases are more common in diabetic patients and the presence of diarrhoea in a diabetic patient should raise the suspicion of coeliac disease, especially if there is coexisting folate or vitamin B_{12} deficiency. However, in the work-up of the diabetic patient with diarrhoea, investigations should first be aimed at isolating any discreet cause. Initially whether or not there is true diarrhoea needs to be established. A 3 day faecal collection allows assessment of volume (normal <200 g/day) and fat content (normal <3 g/day). Upper GI endoscopy with duodenal biopsies will rule out coeliac disease (supported by anti-endomysial antibodies or the more recent tissue transglutaminase levels). As discussed, in the setting of steatorrhea, pancreatic function testing is useful as an adjunct to faecal fat collection. Small bowel bacterial overgrowth should be looked for, preferably with a test such as the C^{14}-xylose test (as discussed), although jejunal aspiration and culture remains the gold standard. Colonoscopy with biopsies will look for evidence of microscopic colitis and allow mucosal assessment and biopsy for inflammatory bowel disease. Type 1 diabetes mellitus has been found to be associated with inflammatory bowel disease in some case reports,[101] and microscopic colitis was found to be more common in diabetic patients in a recent large population study.[102]

If no cause can be found and there is documented large-volume diarrhoea, then it is possible that it is secondary to autonomic neuropathy. *In vivo* studies in the streptozotocin rat model of diabetes demonstrated a decrease in sympathetic tone in the ileal and colonic mucosa that resulted in diarrhoea,[103] and an *in vitro* study demonstrated that the impaired sympathetic tone was accompanied by adrenergic-denervation hypersensitivity.[33] Treatment with the α_2-adrenergic agonist clonidine reverses the diarrhoea in a rat model.[33] Clonidine has therefore been used in the treatment of diabetic diarrhoea, which is thought to be secondary to autonomic neuropathy. Its use is limited to some extent by the side effect of orthostatic hypotension, and at high doses of 0.5–0.6 mg per 12 h, the beneficial effects can be outweighed by its sedative effect.[104] It is sensible to start at a low dose (0.5 mg twice daily) and increase slowly if the drug is proving effective and well tolerated.

If clonidine is ineffective then there is some evidence that octreotide may be helpful. However, this must be given parenterally, which limits its use. It probably works by improving small intestinal motility, and its beneficial effects are dose-dependent, in that higher doses can actually be detrimental and produce steator-rhoea.[105,106] A newer orally active variant is available, although no evidence has as yet been published on its efficacy in diabetic diarrhoea. A flow chart for the approach to diabetic diarrhoea is shown in Figure 8.6.

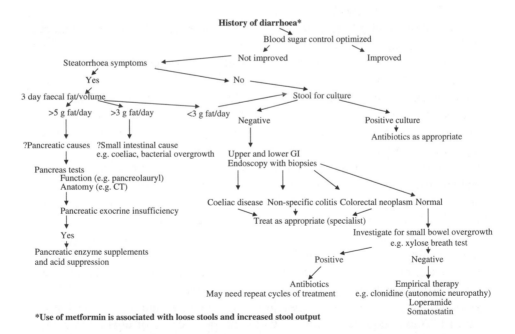

Figure 8.6   Flow chart of the initial investigation of diarrhoea in the diabetic patient

8.13 Conclusion

It has become clear in recent years that GI symptoms are indeed common in the diabetic population and that these symptoms can be associated with physiological abnormalities of the entire GI tract. As with all other complications, tight control of blood sugar is still the most useful intervention, both in terms of prevention of development of complications and in terms of symptom control. The complexity of gut function and the multiple levels at which the gut can be affected in diabetes offers many therapeutic challenges, but with an evolving understanding of the pathophysiology of GI complications in diabetes it is hoped that more specific treatments can be tailored for specific physiological abnormalities.

References

1. Rundles RW. Diabetic neuropathy. *Medicine* 1945; **24**: 111–160.
2. Kassander P. Asymptomatic gastric retention in diabetics: gastroparesis diabeticorum. *Ann Intern Med* 1958; **48**: 797–812.
3. Bytzer P, Talley NJ, Leemon M, Young LJ, Jones MP, Horowitz M. Prevalence of gastrointestinal symptoms associated with diabetes mellitus: a population-based survey of 15,000 adults. *Arch Intern Med* 2001; **161**(16): 1989–1996.
4. Schvarcz E, Palmer M, Ingberg CM, Aman J, Berne C. Increased prevalence of upper gastrointestinal symptoms in long-term type 1 diabetes mellitus. *Diabet Med* 1996; **13**(5): 478–481.
5. Janatuinen E, Pikkarainen P, Laakso M, Pyorala K. Gastrointestinal symptoms in middle-aged diabetic patients. *Scand J Gastroenterol* 1993; **28**(5): 427–432.
6. Enck P, Rathmann W, Spiekermann M, Czerner D, Tschope D, Ziegler D, Strohmeyer G, Gries FA. Prevalence of gastrointestinal symptoms in diabetic patients and non-diabetic subjects. *Z Gastroenterol* 1994; **32**(11): 637–641.
7. Ko GT, Chan WB, Chan JC, Tsang LW, Cockram CS. Gastrointestinal symptoms in Chinese patients with type 2 diabetes mellitus. *Diabet Med* 1999; **16**(8): 670–674.
8. Ricci JA, Siddique R, Stewart WF, Sandler RS, Sloan S, Farup CE. Upper gastrointestinal symptoms in a U.S. national sample of adults with diabetes. *Scand J Gastroenterol* 2000; **35**(2): 152–159.
9. Spangeus A, El Salhy M, Suhr O, Eriksson J, Lithner F. Prevalence of gastrointestinal symptoms in young and middle-aged diabetic patients. *Scand J Gastroenterol* 1999; **34**(12): 1196–1202.
10. Drewes VM. Mechanical and electrical activity in the duodenum of diabetics with and without diarrhea. Pressures, differential pressures and action potentials. *Am J Dig Dis* 1971; **16**(7): 628–634.
11. Whalen GE, Soergel KH, Geenen JE. Diabetic diarrhea. A clinical and pathophysiological study. *Gastroenterology* 1969; **56**(6): 1021–1032.
12. Clouse RE, Lustman PJ. Gastrointestinal symptoms in diabetic patients: lack of association with neuropathy. *Am J Gastroenterol* 1989; **84**(8): 868–872.
13. de Boer SY, Masclee AA, Lamers CB. Effect of hyperglycemia on gastrointestinal and gallbladder motility. *Scand J Gastroenterol Suppl* 1992; **194**: 13–18.
14. Rayner CK, Verhagen MA, Hebbard GS, DiMatteo AC, Doran SM, Horowitz M. Proximal gastric compliance and perception of distension in type 1 diabetes mellitus: effects of hyperglycemia. *Am J Gastroenterol* 2000; **95**(5): 1175–1183.

15. Rayner CK, Samsom M, Jones KL, Horowitz M. Relationships of upper gastrointestinal motor and sensory function with glycemic control. *Diabetes Care* 2001; **24**(2): 371–381.

16. Russo A, Sun WM, Sattawatthamrong Y, Fraser R, Horowitz M, Andrews JM, Read NW. Acute hyperglycaemia affects anorectal motor and sensory function in normal subjects. *Gut* 1997; **41**(4): 494–499.

17. Talley NJ, Hammer J, Giles N, Jones MP, Horowitz M. Measuring gastrointestinal symptoms in diabetes: development and validation of the Diabetes Bowel Symptom Questionnaire. *Gastroenterology* 2001; **120**(suppl 1): A232.

18. Talley NJ, Young L, Bytzer P, Hammer J, Leemon M, Jones M, Horowitz M. Impact of chronic gastrointestinal symptoms in diabetes mellitus on health-related quality of life. *Am J Gastroenterol* 2001; **96**(1): 71–76.

19. Jermendy G, Toth L, Voros P, Koltai MZ, Pogatsa G. Cardiac autonomic neuropathy and QT interval length. A follow-up study in diabetic patients. *Acta Cardiol* 1991; **46**(2): 189–200.

20. Vinik AI, Maser RE, Mitchell BD, Freeman R. Diabetic autonomic neuropathy. *Diabetes Care* 2003; **26**(5): 1553–1579.

21. Yoshida MM, Schuffler MD, Sumi SM. There are no morphologic abnormalities of the gastric wall or abdominal vagus in patients with diabetic gastroparesis. *Gastroenterology* 1988; **94**(4): 907–914.

22. Belai A, Lincoln J, Milner P, Burnstock G. Progressive changes in adrenergic, serotonergic, peptidergic nerves in proximal colon of streptozotocin-diabetic rats. *Gastroenterology* 1988; **95**(5): 1234–1241.

23. Belai A. and Burnstock, G. Changes in adrenergic and peptidergic nerves in the submucous plexus of streptozocin-diabetic rat ileum. *Gastroenterology* 1990; **98**(6): 1427–1436.

24. Belai A, Lefebvre RA, Burnstock G. Motor activity and neurotransmitter release in the gastric fundus of streptozotocin-diabetic rats. *Eur J Pharmac* 1991; **194**(2–3): 225–234.

25. Lincoln J, Bokor JT, Crowe R, Griffith SG, Haven AJ, Burnstock G. Myenteric plexus in streptozotocin-treated rats. Neurochemical and histochemical evidence for diabetic neuropathy in the gut. *Gastroenterology* 1984; **86**(4): 654–661.

26. Soediono P, Belai A, Burnstock G. Prevention of neuropathy in the pyloric sphincter of streptozotocin-diabetic rats by gangliosides. *Gastroenterology* 1993; **104**(4): 1072–1082.

27. Ordog T, Takayama I, Cheung WK, Ward SM, Sanders KM. Remodeling of networks of interstitial cells of Cajal in a murine model of diabetic gastroparesis. *Diabetes* 2000; **49**(10): 1731–1739.

28. He CL, Soffer EE, Ferris CD, Walsh RM, Szurszewski JH, Farrugia G. Loss of interstitial cells of cajal and inhibitory innervation in insulin-dependent diabetes. *Gastroenterology* 2001; **121**(2): 427–434.

29. Watkins CC, Sawa A, Jaffrey S, Blackshaw S, Barrow RK, Snyder SH, Ferris CD. Insulin restores neuronal nitric oxide synthase expression and function that is lost in diabetic gastropathy. *J Clin Invest* 2000; **106**(3): 373–384.

30. Buysschaert M, Donckier J, Dive A, Ketelslegers JM, Lambert AE. Gastric acid and pancreatic polypeptide responses to sham feeding are impaired in diabetic subjects with autonomic neuropathy. *Diabetes* 1985; **34**(11): 1181–1185.

31. Camilleri M. and Malagelada JR. Abnormal intestinal motility in diabetics with the gastroparesis syndrome. *Eur J Clin Invest* 1984; **14**(6): 420–427.

32. Battle WM, Snape WJ. Jr, Alavi A, Cohen S, Braunstein S. Colonic dysfunction in diabetes mellitus. *Gastroenterology* 1980; **79**(6): 1217–1221.

33. Chang EB, Fedorak RN, Field M. Experimental diabetic diarrhea in rats. Intestinal mucosal denervation hypersensitivity and treatment with clonidine. *Gastroenterology* 1986; **91**(3): 564–569.

34. Neil HA, Thompson AV, John S, McCarthy ST, Mann JI. Diabetic autonomic neuropathy: the prevalence of impaired heart rate variability in a geographically defined population. *Diabet Med* 1989; **6**(1): 20–24.

35. Ziegler D, Gries FA, Spuler M, Lessmann F. The epidemiology of diabetic neuropathy. DiaCAN Multicenter Study Group. *Diabet Med* 1993; **10**(suppl 2): 82S–86S.

36. Aziz Q, Thompson DG, Ng VW, Hamdy S, Sarkar S, Brammer MJ, Bullmore ET, Hobson A, Tracey I, Gregory L, Simmons A, Williams SC. Cortical processing of human somatic and visceral sensation. *J Neurosci* 2000; **20**(7): 2657–2663.

37. Emmanuel AV, Kamm MA. Laser Doppler flowmetry as a measure of extrinsic colonic innervation in functional bowel disease. *Gut* 2000; **46**(2): 212–217.

38. Rosenthal JM, Amiel SA, Yaguez L, Bullmore E, Hopkins D, Evans M, Pernet A, Reid H, Giampietro V, Andrew CM, Suckling J, Simmons A, Williams SC. The effect of acute hypoglycemia on brain function and activation: a functional magnetic resonance imaging study. *Diabetes* 2001; **50**(7): 1618–1626.

39. Ferguson SC, Blane A, Perros P, McCrimmon RJ, Best JJ, Wardlaw J, Deary IJ, Frier BM. Cognitive ability and brain structure in type 1 diabetes: relation to microangiopathy and preceding severe hypoglycemia. *Diabetes* 2003; **52**(1): 149–156.

40. Keshavarzian A, Iber FL, Nasrallah S. Radionuclide esophageal emptying and manometric studies in diabetes mellitus. *Am J Gastroenterol* 1987; **82**(7): 625–631.

41. Stewart IM, Hosking DJ, Preston BJ, Atkinson M. Oesophageal motor changes in diabetes mellitus. *Thorax* 1976; **31**(3): 278–283.

42. Kristensson K, Nordborg C, Olsson Y, Sourander P. Changes in the vagus nerve in diabetes mellitus. *Acta Pathol Microbiol Scand A* 1971; **79**(6): 684–685.

43. Rayner CK, Smout AJ, Sun WM, Russo A, Semmler J, Sattawatthamrong Y, Tellis N, Horowitz M. Effects of hyperglycemia on cortical response to esophageal distension in normal subjects. *Dig Dis Sci* 1999; **44**(2): 279–285.

44. Murray FE, Lombard MG, Ashe J, Lynch D, Drury MI, O'Moore B, Lennon J, Crowe J. Esophageal function in diabetes mellitus with special reference to acid studies and relationship to peripheral neuropathy. *Am J Gastroenterol* 1987; **82**(9): 840–843.

45. Clouse RE, Lustman PJ, Reidel WL. Correlation of esophageal motility abnormalities with neuropsychiatric status in diabetics. *Gastroenterology* 1986; **90**(5 Pt 1): 1146–1154.

46. de Caestecker JS, Ewing DJ, Tothill P, Clarke BF, Heading RC. Evaluation of oral cisapride and metoclopramide in diabetic autonomic neuropathy: an eight-week double-blind cross-over study. *Aliment Pharmac Ther* 1989; **3**(1): 69–81.

47. Jones KL, Russo A, Stevens JE, Wishart JM, Berry MK, Horowitz M. Predictors of delayed gastric emptying in diabetes. *Diabetes Care* 2001; **24**(7): 1264–1269.

48. Ziegler D, Schadewaldt P, Pour MA, Piolot R, Schommartz B, Reinhardt M, Vosberg H, Brosicke H, Gries FA. [^{13}C]octanoic acid breath test for non-invasive assessment of gastric emptying in diabetic patients: validation and relationship to gastric symptoms and cardiovascular autonomic function. *Diabetologia* 1996; **39**(7): 823–830.

49. Jones KL, Russo A, Berry MK, Stevens JE, Wishart JM, Horowitz M. A longitudinal study of gastric emptying and upper gastrointestinal symptoms in patients with diabetes mellitus. *Am J Med* 2002; **113**(6): 449–455.

50. Malagelada JR, Rees WD, Mazzotta LJ, Go VL. Gastric motor abnormalities in diabetic and postvagotomy gastroparesis: effect of metoclopramide and bethanechol. *Gastroenterology* 1980; **78**(2): 286–293.

51. Jackson MW, Gordon TP, Waterman SA. Disruption of intestinal motility by a calcium channel-stimulating autoantibody in type 1 diabetes. *Gastroenterology* 2004; **126**(3): 819–828.

52. Samsom M, Akkermans LM, Jebbink RJ, van Isselt H, vanBerge-Henegouwen GP, Smout AJ. Gastrointestinal motor mechanisms in hyperglycaemia induced delayed gastric emptying in type I diabetes mellitus. *Gut* 1997; **40**(5): 641–646.

53. Rayner CK, MacIntosh CG, Chapman IM, Morley JE, Horowitz M. Effects of age on proximal gastric motor and sensory function. *Scand J Gastroenterol* 2000; **35**(10): 1041–1047.

54. Rayner CK, Su YC, Doran SM, Jones KL, Malbert CH, Horowitz M. The stimulation of antral motility by erythromycin is attenuated by hyperglycemia. *Am J Gastroenterol* 2000; **95**(9): 2233–2241.

55. De Boer, SY, Masclee AA, Lam WF, Lemkes HH, Schipper J, Frohlich M, Jansen JB, Lamers CB. Effect of hyperglycaemia on gallbladder motility in type 1 (insulin-dependent) diabetes mellitus. *Diabetologia* 1994; **37**(1): 75–81.

56. Lee JS, Camilleri M, Zinsmeister AR, Burton DD, Choi MG, Nair KS, Verlinden M. Toward office-based measurement of gastric emptying in symptomatic diabetics using [13C]octanoic acid breath test. *Am J Gastroenterol* 2000; **95**(10): 2751–2761.

57. Sturm A, Holtmann G, Goebell H, Gerken G. Prokinetics in patients with gastroparesis: a systematic analysis. *Digestion* 1999; **60**(5): 422–427.

58. Peeters T, Matthijs G, Depoortere I, Cachet T, Hoogmartens J, Vantrappen G. Erythromycin is a motilin receptor agonist. *Am J Physiol* 1989; **257**(3 Pt 1): G470–G474.

59. Janssens J, Peeters TL, Vantrappen G, Tack J, Urbain JL, De Roo M, Muls E, Bouillon R. Improvement of gastric emptying in diabetic gastroparesis by erythromycin. Preliminary studies. *New Engl J Med* 1990; **322**(15): 1028–1031.

60. Fang JC, McCallum RW, DiBaise JK, Schmitt CM, Kipnes MS. Effect of mitemcinal fumarate (GM-611) on gastric emptying in patients with idiopathic or diabetic gastroparesis. *Gastroenterology* 2004; **126**(4 suppl. 2): A483.

61. Ishii M, Nakamura T, Kasai F, Baba T, Takebe K. Erythromycin derivative improves gastric emptying and insulin requirement in diabetic patients with gastroparesis. *Diabetes Care* 1997; **20**(7): 1134–1137.

62. Talley NJ, Verlinden M, Geenen DJ, Hogan RB, Riff D, McCallum RW, Mack RJ. Effects of a motilin receptor agonist (ABT-229) on upper gastrointestinal symptoms in type 1 diabetes mellitus: a randomised, double blind, placebo controlled trial. *Gut* 2001; **49**(3): 395–401.

63. Ehrenpreis ED, Zaitman D, Nellans H. Which form of erythromycin should be used to treat gastroparesis? A pharmacokinetic analysis. *Aliment Pharmac Ther* 1998; **12**(4): 373–376.

64. Abell TL, Van Cutsem E, Abrahamsson H, Huizinga JD, Konturek JW, Galmiche JP, Voeller G, Filez L, Everts B, Waterfall WE, Domschke W, Bruley DV, Familoni BO, Bourgeois IM, Janssens J, Tougas G. Gastric electrical stimulation in intractable symptomatic gastroparesis. *Digestion* 2002; **66**(4): 204–212.

65. Watkins PJ, Buxton-Thomas MS, Howard ER. Long-term outcome after gastrectomy for intractable diabetic gastroparesis. *Diabet Med* 2003; **20**(1): 58–63.

66. Ezzeddine D, Jit R, Katz N, Gopalswamy N, Bhutani MS. Pyloric injection of botulinum toxin for treatment of diabetic gastroparesis. *Gastrointest Endosc* 2002; **55**(7): 920–923.

67. Israel DM, Mahdi G, Hassall E. Pyloric balloon dilation for delayed gastric emptying in children. *Can J Gastroenterol* 2001; **15**(11): 723–727.

68. Masuda Y, Tanaka T, Inomata N, Ohnuma N, Tanaka S, Itoh Z, Hosoda H, Kojima M, Kangawa K. Ghrelin stimulates gastric acid secretion and motility in rats. *Biochem Biophys Res Commun* 2000; **276**(3): 905–908.

69. Murray C, Dass N, Emmanuel A, Sanger G. Facilitation by ghrelin and metoclopramide of nerve-mediated excitatory responses in mouse gastric fundus circular muscle. *Br J Pharmacol* 2002; **136**: 18P.

70. Wegener M, Borsch G, Schaffstein J, Luerweg C, Leverkus F. Gastrointestinal transit disorders in patients with insulin-treated diabetes mellitus. *Dig Dis* 1990; **8**(1): 23–36.

71. Chandalia M, Garg A, Lutjohann D, von Bergmann K, Grundy SM, Brinkley LJ. Beneficial effects of high dietary fiber intake in patients with type 2 diabetes mellitus. *New Engl J Med* 2000; **342**(19): 1392–1398.

72. Giacco R, Parillo M, Rivellese AA, Lasorella G, Giacco A, D'Episcopo L, Riccardi G. Long-term dietary treatment with increased amounts of fiber-rich low-glycemic index natural foods improves blood glucose control and reduces the number of hypoglycemic events in type 1 diabetic patients. *Diabetes Care* 2000; **23**(10): 1461–1466.

73. Russo A, Fraser R, Horowitz M. The effect of acute hyperglycaemia on small intestinal motility in normal subjects. *Diabetologia* 1996; **39**(8): 984–989.

74. Lingenfelser T, Sun W, Hebbard GS, Dent J, Horowitz M. Effects of duodenal distension on antropyloroduodenal pressures and perception are modified by hyperglycemia. *Am J Physiol* 1999; **276**(3 Pt 1): G711–G718.

75. Singh VV, Toskes PP. Small bowel bacterial overgrowth: presentation, diagnosis, treatment. *Curr Gastroenterol Rep* 2003; **5**(5): 365–372.

76. Rolfe RD. The role of probiotic cultures in the control of gastrointestinal health. *J Nutr* 2000; **130**(2S, suppl): 396S–402S.

77. Madrid AM, Hurtado C, Venegas M, Cumsille F, Defilippi C. Long-Term treatment with cisapride and antibiotics in liver cirrhosis: effect on small intestinal motility, bacterial overgrowth, liver function. *Am J Gastroenterol* 2001; **96**(4): 1251–1255.

78. Shanahan F, McKenna R, McCarthy CF, Drury MI. Coeliac disease and diabetes mellitus: a study of 24 patients with HLA typing. *Q J Med* 1982; **51**(203): 329–335.

79. Tesei N, Sugai E, Vazquez H, Smecuol E, Niveloni S, Mazure R, Moreno ML, Gomez JC, Maurino E, Bai JC. Antibodies to human recombinant tissue transglutaminase may detect coeliac disease patients undiagnosed by endomysial antibodies. *Aliment Pharmac Ther* 2003; **17**(11): 1415–1423.

80. Maleki D, Locke GR, III, Camilleri M, Zinsmeister AR, Yawn BP, Leibson C, Melton LJ III. Gastrointestinal tract symptoms among persons with diabetes mellitus in the community. *Arch Intern Med* 2000; **160**(18): 2808–2816.

81. Wald A, Tunuguntla AK. Anorectal sensorimotor dysfunction in fecal incontinence and diabetes mellitus. Modification with biofeedback therapy. *New Engl J Med* 1984; **310**(20): 1282–1287.

82. Russo A, Botten R, Kong MF, Chapman IM, Fraser RJ, Horowitz M, Sun WM. Effects of acute hyperglycaemia on anorectal motor and sensory function in diabetes mellitus. *Diabet Med* 2004; **21**(2): 176–182.

83. Wideroff L, Gridley G, Mellemkjaer L, Chow WH, Linet M, Keehn S, Borch-Johnsen K, Olsen JH. Cancer incidence in a population-based cohort of patients hospitalized with diabetes mellitus in Denmark. *J Natl Cancer Inst* 1997; **89**(18): 1360–1365.

84. Chowdhury RS, Forsmark CE. Review article: pancreatic function testing, *Aliment Pharmac Ther* 2003; **17**(6): 733–750.

85. Nunes AC, Pontes JM, Rosa A, Gomes L, Carvalheiro M, Freitas D. Screening for pancreatic exocrine insufficiency in patients with diabetes mellitus. *Am J Gastroenterol* 2003; **98**(12): 2672–2675.

86. Chowdhury RS, Forsmark CE. Review article: pancreatic function testing. *Aliment Pharmac Ther* 2003; **17**(6): 733–750.

87. Heijerman HG, Lamers CB, Bakker W. Omeprazole enhances the efficacy of pancreatin (pancrease) in cystic fibrosis. *Ann Intern Med* 1991; **114**(3): 200–201.

88. Heijerman HG, Lamers CB, Dijkman JH, Bakker W. Ranitidine compared with the dimethylprostaglandin E2 analogue enprostil as adjunct to pancreatic enzyme replacement in adult cystic fibrosis. *Scand J Gastroenterol Suppl* 1990; **178**: 26–31.

89. Clark JM, Brancati FL, Diehl AM. Nonalcoholic fatty liver disease. *Gastroenterology* 2002; **122**(6): 1649–1657.
90. Jacobs JE, Birnbaum BA, Shapiro MA, Langlotz CP, Slosman F, Rubesin SE, Horii SC. Diagnostic criteria for fatty infiltration of the liver on contrast-enhanced helical CT. *AJR Am J Roentgenol* 1998; **171**(3): 659–664.
91. Laurin J, Lindor KD, Crippin JS, Gossard A, Gores GJ, Ludwig J, Rakela J, McGill DB. Ursodeoxycholic acid or clofibrate in the treatment of non-alcohol-induced steatohepatitis: a pilot study. *Hepatology* 1996; **23**(6): 1464–1467.
92. Horlander JC, Kwo PY, Cummings OW. Atorvastatin for the treatment of NASH. *Gastroenterology* 2001; **120**: A544.
93. Marchesini G, Brizi M, Bianchi G, Tomassetti S, Zoli M, Melchionda N. Metformin in non-alcoholic steatohepatitis. *Lancet* 2001; **358**(9285): 893–894.
94. Krentz AJ, Bailey CJ, Melander A. Thiazolidinediones for type 2 diabetes. New agents reduce insulin resistance but need long term clinical trials. *Br Med J* 2000; **321**(7256): 252–253.
95. Lindor KD, Kowdley KV, Heathcote EJ, Harrison ME, Jorgensen R, Angulo P, Lymp JF, Burgart L, Colin P. Ursodeoxycholic acid for treatment of nonalcoholic steatohepatitis: results of a randomized trial. *Hepatology* 2004; **39**(3): 770–778.
96. El Serag HB, Tran T, Everhart JE. Diabetes increases the risk of chronic liver disease and hepatocellular carcinoma. *Gastroenterology* 2004; **126**(2): 460–468.
97. Mundth ED. Cholecystitis and diabetes mellitus. *New Engl J Med* 1962; **267**: 642–646.
98. Fiorucci S, Bosso R, Scionti L, DiSanto S, Annibale B, Delle FG, Morelli A. Neurohumoral control of gallbladder motility in healthy subjects and diabetic patients with or without autonomic neuropathy. *Dig Dis Sci* 1990; **35**(9): 1089–1097.
99. Hahm JS, Park JY, Park KG, Ahn YH, Lee MH, Park KN. Gallbladder motility in diabetes mellitus using real time ultrasonography. *Am J Gastroenterol* 1996; **91**(11): 2391–2394.
100. de Boer SY, Masclee AA, Lam WF, Lemkes HH, Schipper J, Frohlich M, Jansen JB, Lamers CB. Effect of hyperglycaemia on gallbladder motility in type 1 (insulin-dependent) diabetes mellitus. *Diabetologia* 1994; **37**(1): 75–81.
101. Kay M, Wyllie R, Michener W, Caulfield M, Steffen R. Associated ulcerative colitis, sclerosing cholangitis, insulin-dependent diabetes mellitus. *Cleve Clin J Med* 1993; Nov–Dec: 473–478.
102. Olesen M, Eriksson S, Bohr J, Jarnerot G, Tysk C. Lymphocytic colitis: a retrospective clinical study of 199 Swedish patients. *Gut* 2004; 536–541.
103. Chang EB, Bergenstal RM, Field M. Diarrhea in streptozocin-treated rats. Loss of adrenergic regulation of intestinal fluid and electrolyte transport. *J Clin Invest* 1985; **75**(5): 1666–1670.
104. Fedorak RN, Field M, Chang EB. Treatment of diabetic diarrhea with clonidine. *Ann Intern Med* 1985; **102**(2): 197–199.
105. Tsai ST, Vinik AI, Brunner JF. Diabetic diarrhea and somatostatin. *Ann Intern Med* 1986; **104**(6): 894.
106. Witt K, Pedersen NT. The long-acting somatostatin analogue SMS 201–995 causes malabsorption. *Scand J Gastroenterol* 1989; **24**(10): 1248–1252.

9

Diabetes and Musculoskeletal Disease

D. L. Browne and F. C. McCrae

9.1 Introduction

Vascular complication is the principal cause of morbidity and mortality in diabetes, yet it is often forgotten that diabetes is a multisystemic disease affecting all organs, including musculoskeletal tissue. Despite the increased prevalence of musculoskeletal disorders amongst the diabetic population, this area is frequently neglected in the clinic setting. Musculoskeletal disease reduces functional ability, quality of life and exercise capacity in diabetic patients already suffering from reduced health status. Consequent reduced exercise capacity predisposes the diabetic patient to weight gain and increased vascular risk.

This chapter reviews current understanding regarding the musculoskeletal complications of diabetes and their relevance to the diabetic individual *per se*.

Certain connective tissue diseases such as cheiroarthropathy are associated almost exclusively with diabetes, whilst others such as Dupuytren's and carpal tunnel disease merely occur more frequently in the diabetic population. The pathophysiological of the musculoskeletal complications of diabetes are examined prior to review of the individual conditions associated with diabetes

9.2 Pathophysiology

The pathophysiological explanations for musculoskeletal complications of diabetes are diffuse and understanding remains incomplete (Table 9.1). The mechanisms

Diabetes: Chronic Complications   Edited by Kenneth M. Shaw and Michael H. Cummings
© 2005 John Wiley & Sons, Ltd.

Table 9.1 Potential mechanisms for increased incidence of musculoskeletal disease in diabetes

Consequences of chronic hyperglycaemia

Glycosylation of connective tissue
Increased connective tissue deposition due to proliferation of myofibroblasts
Increased basal inflammatory tone

Consequences of diabetic complications

Neuropathy
Vascular insufficiency

Consequences of conditions associated with diabetes

Autoimmune links with type 1 diabetes
Abnormal levels of insulin and insulin-like growth hormone
Obesity

---

leading to increased musculoskeletal disease can be divided into direct consequences of persistent hyperglycaemia, consequences of diabetic complications and consequences of conditions associated with diabetes, including obesity.

Firstly there are the effects of persistent hyperglycaemia on the quality and quantity of connective tissue. Hyperglycaemia stimulates non-enzymatic glycosylation of protein resulting in advanced glycation end product (AGE) formation and connective tissue stiffening.[1] Furthermore, glycosylated collagen is antigenic and can induce an antibody reaction causing further alteration of connective tissue.[2] In addition, the deposition of connective tissue is increased in diabetes, potentially mediated through increased proliferation of myofibroblasts.[1]

Secondly, the vascular insufficiency and neuropathy associated with diabetes increases the risk of osteomyelitis, avascular necrosis and joint destruction (Charcot joints). The aforementioned pathophysiological processes are discussed elsewhere in this textbook.

Thirdly, the consequences of conditions associated with diabetes on the musculoskeletal structure should be considered. There are shared genetic links between type 1 diabetes and other autoimmune diseases such as rheumatoid arthritis.[3] Genetic links between the organ-specific autoimmune conditions (HLA DR3/DR4 tissue antigens) explain the familial clustering of rheumatoid arthritis and type 1 diabetes.[4] Unsubstantiated reports suggest that rheumatoid arthritis is more progressive and affects large joints when accompanied by type 1 diabetes.[5] Moreover, joint surgery in patients with rheumatoid arthritis and co-existing diabetes carries additional risk.

The deficiency of insulin and insulin-like growth factor seen with type 1 diabetes and the hyperinsulinaemia associated with type 2 diabetes may contribute to skeletal anomalies.[6] Insulin stimulates collagen synthesis and influences the proteoglycan composition of bone and cartilage[7] whilst insulin-like growth factors (such as IGF-1) stimulate osteoblast activity.[8]

Finally, the role of obesity and physical inactivity must be considered when discussing musculoskeletal conditions and diabetes. Type 2 diabetes is integrally linked to obesity, physical inactivity and oversupply of calories. The metabolic syndrome is accompanied by an altered secretion pattern of adipokines, produced by adipocytes, which not only alter insulin sensitivity but also inhibit function of skeletal muscle by three mechanisms.[9] Firstly, intramyocellular accumulation of lipids diminishes kinase signalling within the myocytes of obese subjects.[9] Secondly, obesity is associated with augmented basal inflammatory tone, in part originating from elevated adipokine activity, which may be deleterious to muscle. Finally, in obese patients adipocytes accumulate within skeletal muscle itself and exert direct paracrine effects on adjacent myocytes.[9]

In addition to the defects in insulin and adipokines, abnormalities in leptin have also been reported in obese diabetic subjects.[10] Both leptin and insulin modulate the sodium/potassium (Na^+, K^+) pumps which control membrane potential, osmotic balance and consequent cell volume of cardiac and skeletal myocytes. It has been postulated that abnormalities of Na^+, K^+ pump activity contribute to abnormal vascular function in diabetic patients with parallel defects occurring within skeletal muscle.[10]

9.3 Musculoskeletal Conditions Associated with Diabetes

The musculoskeletal conditions most commonly associated with diabetes are discussed below. One or more of the aforementioned pathogenic mechanisms may be implicated in an association of a musculoskeletal condition with diabetes. Some rheumatological conditions are exclusive to diabetes whilst others occur more frequently in the diabetic population compared with non-diabetics. Whilst some musculoskeletal conditions may be managed conventionally when associated with diabetes, others may require special considerations as discussed below. There is a preponderance of rheumatological manifestations of diabetes in the upper limb, although some conditions occur throughout the skeletal system.

9.4 Upper Limb Diabetic Complications

Shoulder adhesive capsulitis

Shoulder adhesive capsulitis presents as shoulder pain associated with generalized reduction of movement, occurring in up to 30 per cent of patients with diabetes[11] compared with 2.5 per cent of the non-diabetic population. The condition is also more commonly bilateral in diabetes. Owing to increased connective tissue production, the joint capsule thickens and adheres to the humoral head with associated inflammation. The condition may persist for several years prior to recovery, but then relapse at a future time. Increasing age and duration of diabetes are associated with shoulder adhesive capsulitis but no clear association has been seen with other complications of diabetes.[11] Treatment of adhesive capsulitis is largely conservative, with physiotherapy and manipulation, although intra-articular steroids have been used.[11]

Shoulder–hand syndrome

Shoulder–hand syndrome (SHS) consists of adhesive capsulitis of the shoulder and painful, swollen, tender hands associated with vasomotor and skin changes. There is a large overlap between SHS and Sudecks atrophy (reflex sympathetic dystrophy) and, if left untreated, permanent loss of function may result. Whilst it is most commonly associated with trauma, one study found that 7.4 per cent of patients with SHS also had diabetes. However, with current diagnostic criteria for diabetes, the prevalence might be higher.[12] Treatment of SHS consists of analgesia and physiotherapy, although sympathetic ganglion block (surgical or guanethidine) may be required, resulting in 80 per cent improvement.[13]

Limited joint mobility

Limited joint mobility (LJM; Figure 9.1), or cheiroarthropathy, is almost exclusively associated with diabetes and involves the small joints of the hand. Patients may complain of stiffness, loss of dexterity and weakness, but cheiroarthropathy is painless. On examination the skin is thickened and tight and the patient may exhibit the 'prayer sign' due to contracture of the flexor tendons. Biopsy of the skin reveals increased collagen deposition. LJM is more important for its associations than its symptoms. The prevalence amongst diabetic populations of LJM varies depending on the method of assessment, but figures above 50 per cent have been reported in type 1[14] and type 2 diabetes.[15] Arkkila[14,15] found LJM to be associated with a 9.3- and 3.3-fold risk of proliferative retinopathy and neuropathy, respectively, in type 2 diabetes, with a similar increased risk amongst type 1 patients. In type 2 patients LJM was also associated with macrovascular disease and suboptimal glycaemic control. Whilst the incidence of LJM tends to increase with duration of diabetes, it may occur soon after diagnosis, particularly amongst adolescents with type 1 diabetes.[16] Treatment of LJM itself is seldom needed, although improvement of glycaemic control should be aimed for, whilst surgery and corticosteroid injection may alleviate severe symptoms.[17]

Dupuytren's disease

Dupuytren's disease consists of focal flexor contracture and a thickened band of palmar fascia of the hand. Whilst it is common in the general population,

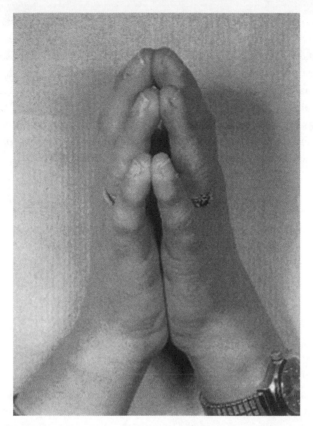

Figure 9.1 The clinical 'prayer sign' due to contracture of the flexor tendons (Reproduced from *Pract Diab Int* (2001) **18**: 63 by permission of John Wiley & Sons, Ltd.)

Dupuytren's occurs more frequently in diabetic patients, with a prevalence approaching 30 per cent.[18] Jennings reported the presence of Dupuytren's to be associated with twice the risk of vision threatening retinopathy and a fivefold increase in the risk of foot ulceration in type 2 diabetes.[18] In type 1 diabetes, the association between Dupuytren's and diabetic complications is less clear following a prospective study which concluded that any association was explained by patient age and duration of diabetes.[19] There is, however, an association between Dupuytren's and other connective tissue disorders such as LJM and shoulder capsulitis in both type 1 and type 2 diabetes.[18] Dupuytren's may be treated either conservatively or surgically depending on the severity, and may recur.

Carpal tunnel syndrome

Carpal tunnel syndrome (CTS) is associated with several conditions including hypothyroidism, but diabetes remains the commonest associated disease, studies suggesting a prevalence of between 15 and 25 per cent amongst diabetic out-patients.[20] CTS presents with paraesthesia of the hand and forearm, typically worse at night, caused by compression of the median nerve by fibrosis, although in diabetes ischaemia of the vasa nervorum may contribute to the development of CTS. Diagnosis is confirmed by nerve conduction studies which differentiate CTS from other diabetic peripheral neuropathy. Correlation between CTS and micro-angiopathy has been noted in diabetes.[20] Treatment of CTS involves wrist splints and surgical decompression. Corticosteroid injections are less helpful in patients with diabetes as the aetiology is usually non-inflammatory.

9.5   Generalized Conditions Involving the Skeletal System in Diabetes

Whilst the connective tissue changes witnessed with diabetes predominantly affect the upper limbs, other abnormalities occur throughout the diabetic skeleton.

Hyperostosis

Diffuse idiopathic skeletal hyperostosis (Forestier's disease) mimics ankylosing spondylitis, but occurs in middle-aged men, particularly those who are obese with type 2 diabetes,[21] although some authors dispute an association with diabetes.[22] Ossification of spinal ligaments and osteophyte formation eventually leads to ankylosing of the vertebrae, with the thoracic spine most often affected. Hyper-insulinaemia has been implicated in the development of Forestier's as insulin may promote new bone growth.[23] The condition is usually asymptomatic but may cause pain and stiffness, although radiological appearances may be more severe.

Diabetic osteopenia

Reduced bone mass (osteopenia) has been widely reported with type 1 diabetes.[24] It has been postulated that the mechanism for 'diabetic osteopathy' is a combina-tion of inflammation-mediated osteopenia and reduced levels of insulin-like growth factor.[7] Insulin and insulin-like growth factor stimulate bone calcification, amino acid incorporation and collagen synthesis. In addition, unexplained abnorm-alities of plasma biochemistry (elevated alkaline phosphatase and decreased vitamin D, parathyroid hormone and calcitonon levels) suggesting abnormal bone metabolism have been reported in patients with type 1 diabetes.[1,25,26]

Progression of diabetic osteopenia has been linked to the presence of retino-pathy,[27] but there is no convincing evidence of an increased incidence of osteoporotic fractures in the diabetic population.[28] In contrast, patients with type 2 diabetes have normal or even increased bone density, possibly due to increased levels of adipose tissue, which produces insulin-related growth factors which stimulate bone growth.[24,28]

Gout, pseudogout and osteoarthritis

Gout is seen more commonly in patients with type 2 diabetes for two reasons.[29] Firstly, hyperuricaemia is associated with insulin resistance even prior to the development of diabetes and would appear to be integral to the metabolic syndrome.[30] Secondly, the vascular burden seen with diabetes results in the widespread use of drugs, such as thiazide diuretics, which predispose to gout. A relationship between chondrocalcinosis and diabetes is less clear, with some authors suggesting no connection,[31] whilst others suggest weak association.[32] Whilst osteoarthritis and type 2 diabetes are both linked and exacerbated by obesity, no association between diabetes and osteoarthritis is found following adjustment for weight.[33] Nevertheless, C-reactive protein, a quantitative marker of the acute phase response linked to atherosclerosis, obesity and diabetes, has also been found to correlate with the development of osteoarthritis of the knee.[34]

Ischaemic, infective and neuropathic processes

A combination of vascular insufficiency, neuropathy, infection and metabolic abnormalities predispose the diabetic patient to the 'diabetic foot'. Whilst discussion of the pathology and management of diabetic foot disease is outside the scope of this chapter, it is important to remember that these processes may also affect other areas of the skeleton.

Widespread microangiopathy is common in patients with long-standing diabetes. Microvascular disease usually presents as retinopathy, nephropathy or neuropathy, but rarely results in skeletal muscle infarction. Clinicians should be alert to the diagnosis of diabetic muscle infarction in patients with established microangiopathy who present with an isolated painful muscle, and T_2-weighted magnetic resonance imaging is valuable in confirming the diagnosis.[35]

The impaired neutrophil function associated with diabetes predisposes patients to haematogenous spread of infection to bones other than the foot. The vertebrae are often affected and unusual causal organisms may be isolated in diabetic patients.[36] When osteomyelitis is suspected in diabetic patients, imaging with MRI, ultrasound and bone scintigraphy should be considered when plain radiographs have been unhelpful.[37]

Charcot's (neuropathic) arthropathy

Neuropathic arthropathy, also known as Charcot joint, was first described in 1868 by Jean Martin Charcot and occurs as a consequence of many diseases in which sensation is impaired, although most commonly in association with diabetes. Diabetic neuroarthropathy predominantly affects the feet (discussed elsewhere in this textbook). However, in association with diabetes, Charcot's joints have also been reported in knees, wrists, elbows, shoulders and intervertebral joints.[38] Neuropathic arthropathy should be considered in a patient with long-standing diabetes and sensory impairment complaining of an unexplained swollen joint. It has been suggested that autonomic neuropathy is involved in the pathophysiology of diabetic neuroarthropathy. Impaired autonomic innervation stimulates local blood flow resulting in augmented bone resorption, leading to osteoporosis, fractures and joint damage.[39]

9.6   Functional Disability in Diabetic Patients

The socio-economic burden of diabetes is exploding throughout the developed world. Not only is the prevalence of diabetes increasing but diagnosis is occurring at a younger age. Whilst macrovascular disease is the predominant cause of disability amongst patients with diabetes, the contribution of non-vascular functional impairment should not be overlooked. A wide variety of non-vascular factors predispose diabetic patients to reduced mobility and function with consequent dependence and tendency to weight gain (Table 9.2).

Table 9.2   Factors resulting in reduced physical function in diabetes

Macrovascular disease, e.g. cerebrovascular accident (CVA), amputations
Painful neuropathy
Foot ulceration
Musculoskeletal complications of diabetes
Obesity
Fibromyalgia
Disorders of balance
Muscle infarction, infection and inflammation
Psychological, e.g. depression, fear of exercise-induced hypoglycaemia

An epidemiological study has shown patients with diabetes to be at increased risk of posterior semicircular canal benign paroxysmal vertigo (BPV) and impaired balance as measured by computerized dynamic posturography.[40] The aetiology of the increased vestibular disease in diabetic subjects has not been established, nor the prevalence of BPV in the diabetic population.

Patients with diabetes are prescribed an increasing number of medications to combat hyperglycaemia and associated vascular risk factors and complications. Whilst medications such as statins are well recognized to cause muscular symptoms, it is often forgotten that frequently reported adverse events of oral hypoglycaemic agents include musculoskeletal complications.[41]

Whilst the pathophysiology of fibromyalgia is poorly understood, the condition can be associated with significant functional limitation. Several studies have reported high levels of fibromyalgia in diabetic subjects. In Italian diabetic patients diffuse musculoskeletal pain in 62 per cent of patients with type 2 diabetes and obesity was found to be an independent risk factor.[42] A further study demonstrated no increased prevalence of fibromyalgia in diabetic men, but significantly higher rates of fibromyalgia amongst women with diabetes.[43] Furthermore, severity of fibromyalgia correlates with the duration of diabetes.[43]

9.7 Conclusion

Both type 1 and type 2 diabetes are associated with an increased prevalence of joint and connective tissue diseases. Further investigation of the rheumatological manifestations of diabetes is required as to date most evidence comes from small epidemiological studies. In addition to causing significant morbidity there is evidence that certain conditions, such as cheiroarthropathy, may be markers of microvascular risk. There is therefore a rationale for including a musculoskeletal survey in the diabetic consultation.

References

1. Rosenbloom AL, Silverstein JH. Connective tissue and joint disease in diabetes mellitus. *Endocrinol Metab Clin N Am* 1996; **25**(2): 473–483.
2. Bassiouny AR, Rosenberg H, McDonald TL. Glycosylated collagen is antigenic. *Diabetes* 1983; **32**: 1181–1184.
3. Vaidya B, Imrie H, Perros P, Young ET, Kelly WF, Carr D, Large DM, Toft AD, Kendall-Taylor P, Pearce SH. Evidence for a new Graves disease susceptibility locus at chromosome 18q21. *Am J Hum Genet* 2000; **66**(5): 1710–1714.
4. Thomas DJ, Young A, Gorsuch AN, Bottazzo GF, Cudworth AG. Evidence for an association between rheumatoid arthritis and autoimmune endocrine disease. *Ann Rheum Dis* 1983; **42**: 297–300.
5. Forgacs S. *Bones and Joints in Diabetes Mellitus*. Nijhoff: The Hague, 1992.
6. Kemink SA, Hermus AR, Swinkels LM, Lutterman JA, Smals AG. Osteopenia in insulin-dependent diabetes mellitus; prevalence and aspects of pathophysiology. *J Endocrinol Invest* 2000; **23**(5): 295–303.
7. Weiss R, Gorn A, Nimmi M. Abnormalities in the biosynthesis of cartilage and bone proteoglycans in experimental diabetes. *Diabetes* 1981 Aug; **30**(8): 670–7.
8. Canalis E. Bone related growth factors. *Triangle* 1988; **27**: 11–19.
9. Nawrocki AR, Scherer PE. The delicate balance between fat and muscle: adipokines in metabolic disease and musculoskeletal inflammation. *Curr Opin Pharmac* 2004; **4**(3): 281–289.

10. Sweeney G, Klip A. Mechanisms and consequences of Na^+, K^+-pump regulation by insulin and leptin. *Cell Mol Biol* (*Noisy-le-grand*) 2001; **47**(2): 363–372.
11. Balci N, Balci MK, Tuzuner S. Shoulder capsulitis and shoulder range of motion in type II diabetes mellitus: association with diabetic complications. *J Diabet Complic* 1999; **13**(3): 135–140.
12. Doury P, Dirheimer Y, Pattin S. *Algodystrophy: Diagnosis and Therapy of a Frequent Disease of the Locomotor Apparatus.* Springer: Berlin, 1981.
13. Steinbroker O, Argyros TG. The shoulder–hand syndrome: present status as a diagnostic and therapeutic entity. *Med Clin N Am* 1958; **42**: 1533–1553.
14. Arkkila PE, Kantola IM, Viikari JS. Limited joint mobility in type 1 diabetic patients: correlation to other complications. *J Intern Med* 1994; **236**(2): 215–216.
15. Arkkila PE, Kantola IM, Viikari JS. Limited joint mobility in non-insulin-dependent diabetic patients: correlation to control of diabetes, atherosclerotic vascular disease, and other diabetic complications. *J Diabetes Complic* 1997; **11**(4): 208–217.
16. Clarke CF, Piesowicz AT, Spathis GS. Limited joint mobility in children and adolescents with insulin dependent diabetes mellitus. *Ann Rheum Dis* 1990; **49**(4): 236–237.
17. Aljahlan M, Lee KC, Toth E. Limited joint mobility in diabetes. *Postgrad Med* 1999; **105**(2): 99–101, 105–106.
18. Jennings AM, Milner PC, Ward JD. Hand abnormalities are associated with the complications of diabetes in type 2 diabetes. *Diabet Med* 1989; **6**(1): 43–47.
19. Arkkila PE, Kantola IM, Viikari JS, Ronnemaa T, Vahatalo MA. Dupuytren's disease in type 1 diabetic patients: a five-year prospective study. *Clin Exp Rheumatol* 1996; **14**(1): 59–65.
20. Chammas M, Bousquet P, Renard E, Poirier JL, Jaffiol C, Allieu Y. Dupuytren's disease, carpal tunnel syndrome, trigger finger, and diabetes mellitus. *J Hand Surg* 1995; **20**(1): 109–114.
21. Julkunen H, Heinonen OP, Kinekt P, Maatela J. The epidemiology of hyperostosis of the spine together with its symptoms and related mortality in ageneral population. *Scand J Rheum* 1975; **4**: 23–27.
22. Traillet N, Gerster J-C. Forestier's disease and metabolic disorders. A prospective controlled study of 25 cases. *Rev Rheum* 1993; **60**: 274–279.
23. Littlejohn G. Insulin and new bone formation in diffuse idiopathic skeletal hyperostosis. *Clin Rheum* 1985; **4**: 294–300.
24. Zeigler R. Diabetes mellitus and bone metabolism. *Horm Metab Res Suppl* 1992; **26**: 90–94.
25. Frazer TE, White NH, Hough S. Alterations in circulating vitamin D metabolites in the young insulin dependent diabetic. *J Clin Endocrinol Metab* 1981; **53**: 1154–1159.
26. McNair P, Christiansen MS, Madsbad S. Hypoparathyroidism in diabetes mellitus. *Acta Endocrinol* 1981; **96**: 81–86.
27. Campos Pastor MM, Lopez-Ibarra PJ, Escobar-Jimenez F, Serrano Pa MD, Garcia-Cervigon AG. Intensive insulin therapy and bone mineral density in type 1 diabetes mellitus: a prospective study. *Osteoporosis Int* 2000; **11**(5): 455–459.
28. Piepkorn B, Kann P, Forst T, Andreas J, Pfutzner A, Beyer J. Bone mineral density and bone metabolism in diabetes mellitus. *Horm Metab Res* 1997; **29**(11): 584–591.
29. Mitchell P, Smith W, Wang JJ, Cumming RG, Leeder SR, Burnett L. Diabetes in older Australian population. *Diabetes Res Clin Pract* 1998; **41**(3): 177–184.
30. Kekalainen P, Sarlund H, Laakso M. Long-term association of cardiovascular risk factors with increased insulin secretion and insulin resistance. *Metabolism* 2000; **49**(10): 1247–1254.
31. Silveri F, Adamo V, Corsi M, Brecciaroli D, Pettinari P, Urbani C, Carotti A, Cervini C. Chondrocalcinosis an diabetes mellitus. The clinico-statistical data. *Rec Prog Med* 1994; **85**(2): 91–95.

32. Baba H, Maezawa Y, Kawahara N, Tomita K, Furusawa N, Imura S. Calcium crystal deposition in the ligamentum flavum of the spine. *Spine* 1993; **18**(15): 2174–2181.

33. Frey MI, Barrett-Connor E, Sledge PA, Schneider DL, Weisman MH. The effect of non-insulin dependent diabetes mellitus on the prevalence of clinical osteoarthritis. A population based study. *J Rheumatol* 1996; **23**(4): 716–722.

34. Sowers M, Jannausch M, Stein E, Jamadar D, Hochberg M, Lachance L. C-reactive protein as a biomarker of emergent osteoarthritis. *Osteoarthrit Cart* 2002; **10**(8): 595–601.

35. Chow KM, Szeto CC, Griffith JF, Wong TY, Li PK. Unusual muscle pain in two patients with diabetic renal failure. *Hong Kong Med J* 2002; **8**(5): 368–371.

36. Solis-Garcia del Pozo J, Martinez-Alfaro E, Abad L, Solero J. Vertebral osteomyelitis caused by *Streptococcus agalactiae*. *J Infect* 2000; **41**(1): 84–90.

37. Becker W. Imaging osteomyelitis and the diabetic foot. *Q J Nucl Med* 1999; **43**(1): 9–20.

38. Sinha S, Munichoodappa CS, Kozak GP. Neuroarthropathy in diabetes mellitus. *Medicine* 1972; **51**: 191–210.

39. Brower AC, Allman RM. Pathogenesis of the neuropathic joint: neurotraumatic vs neurovascular. *Radiology* 1981; **139**: 349–354.

40. Cohen HS, Kimball KT, Stewart MG. Benign paroxysmal positional vertigo and comorbid conditions. *ORL H Otorhinolaryngol Relat Spec* 2004; **66**(1): 11–15.

41. Plosker GL. Figgitt DP. Repaglinide: a pharmacoeconomic review of its use in type 2 diabetes mellitus. *Pharmacoeconomics* 2004; **22**(6): 389–411.

42. Patucchi E, Fatati G, Puxeddu A, Coaccioli S. Prevalence of fibromyalgia in diabetes mellitus and obesity. *Rec Prog Med* 2003; **94**(4): 163–165.

43. Wolak T, Weizman S, Harman-Boehm I, Friger M, Sukenik S. Prevalence of fibromyalgia in type 2 diabetes mellitus. *Harefuah* 2001; **140**(11): 1006–1009, 1119, 1120.

10

Diabetes and the Skin

Adam Haworth

10.1 Introduction

For the diabetic patient, skin disease is rarely life-threatening but often causes significant distress due to its appearance, itching and ulceration. It also can act as an important marker of complications in other systems. This chapter discusses the various disorders that can be seen in the skin of diabetic patients and details the steps necessary in confirming the diagnosis, possible complications and treatments that are available to non-dermatologists and likely treatments after a dermatological referral. Short notes will be provided on specialist dermatology treatments for further information. As with diabetic complications in other systems, many of the pathological changes are due to microangiopathy and also the non-enzymatic glycosylation (NEG) of proteins, in particular collagen. This section will discuss the histiocytic response conditions, granuloma annulare and necrobiosis lipoidica, the diabetic thick skin conditions related to NEG of collagen, acanthosis nigricans secondary to hyperinsulinaemia, some of the infections that can be more prevalent in diabetic patients and the rarer diabetic dermopathy, perforating disorders and bullosis diabeticorum. Diabetic ulceration is covered elsewhere in Chapter 3. At the end of the chapter are two sections, one reviewing the dermatological vocabulary used by dermatologists in an attempt to maintain the mystique around our subject and the other outlining the dermatological therapies that may not be familiar to non-dermatologists.

Diabetes: Chronic Complications   Edited by Kenneth M. Shaw and Michael H. Cummings
© 2005 John Wiley & Sons, Ltd.

10.2   Necrobiotic Disorders

Granuloma annulare and necrobiosis lipoidica (diabeticorum) are both disorders that show a histiocytic response to a region of destruction of collagen and elastin. Histologically they are very similar, with a central area of necrobiotic collagen (partial necrosis giving a fragmented and altered appearance) surrounded by lymphocytes and a cuff of histiocytes. This is a typical granulomatous or "foreign body" reaction. The difference between the two conditions is in the amount of necrosis and the changes tend to occur in small foci in granuloma annulare, representing each papule seen on the skin, whilst in necrobiosis they occur in sheets with more atrophy, hence being able to see fat through the atrophied skin, giving a yellow, lipoid appearance. The histological features can be very subtle and difficult to find in a biopsy specimen, and differentiating between the two diagnoses and rheumatoid nodules, which have a similar histological appearance, can be extremely difficult. Often one has to be led by the clinical appearance and any histological evidence of necrobiosis. It has been postulated that glycosylation of collagen makes it immunogenic and hence stimulates this foreign body reaction.

Granuloma annulare

Granuloma annulare (GA) typically presents with annular plaques made up of skin-coloured or red/purple papules, most commonly occurring on the hands and feet (Figure 10.1). They are usually asymptomatic but can occasionally itch. The majority of cases will resolve spontaneously and need no treatment, but the main morbidity comes from it being visible on the hands and inappropriately treated,

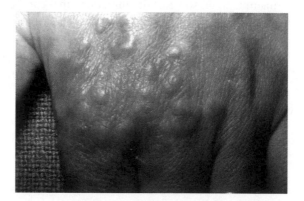

Figure 10.1   Localized granuloma annulare with typical dermal papules over the knuckles. Note that the skin markings are maintained and there is no scale (courtesy of Dr Richard Ashton, Haslar Hospital, Gosport)

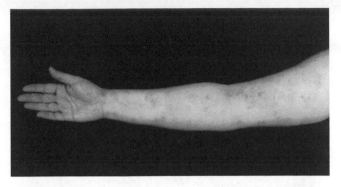

Figure 10.2 Generalized granuloma annulare with multiple less well-defined annular plaques. There is widespread distribution including the trunk. This patient also had necrobiosis lipoidica

usually as a fungal infection. There are five variants, the most common being the annular or localized form (Figure 10.1); generalized GA is rarer but seems to be more closely related to diabetes (Figure 10.2). Papular umbilicated, linear and deep or subcutaneous GA are very rare.

The link of granuloma annulare with diabetes has long been discussed, but is now accepted, particularly for the generalized form. For localized GA the evidence is less strong with studies supporting both sides;[1] however Muhlemann and Williams[2] showed, using age-matched population data in 557 patients with GA, that 16 had insulin-dependent diabetes compared with an expected number for the population of 0.9. Dabski and Winkelmann[3] looked at 100 patients with generalized GA and found that 21 per cent had diabetes; for localized GA this was reduced to 10 per cent.

GA may present at any age but the localized form is more common in young adults and has a female preponderance in all types. Generalized GA is more likely to present later in life and consists of multiple 1–2 mm papules that either form sheets or may be arranged in rings. The trunk is more commonly affected than the limbs, as compared with the annular variant, and the likelihood of spontaneous resolution is less at 8 per cent,[3] with most patients continuing on a remitting and relapsing course.

Differential diagnosis is usually limited as the clinical appearance is characteristic and biopsy is usually only necessary in the generalized form. Granulomatous conditions such as annular sarcoidosis can be difficult but usually have a brown appearance; lichen planus can also have an annular form that can look similar, although more purple. In the annular form GA is often mistaken for and commonly treated as a fungal infection. Being a dermal disease with no disruption of the epidermis, GA has no scale and the fine skin markings can clearly be seen over the ring of papules. The epithelial involvement in *Tinea corporis* (ringworm) gives the annular plaques a peripheral scale and the fine skin markings are disturbed over the advancing edge (Figures 10.3 and 10.4). Where the diagnosis is in

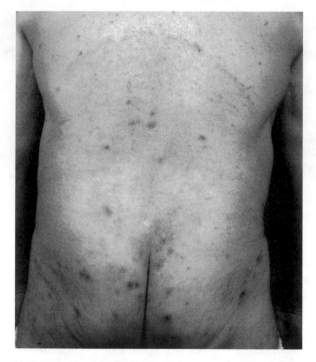

Figure 10.3   Tinea corporis; widespread annulare itchy eruption with a peripheral scale

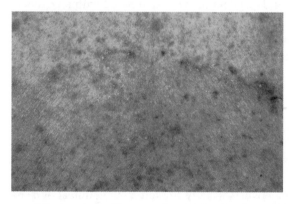

Figure 10.4   Close-up of Figure 10.3 to illustrate the peripheral scale and disruption of the skin markings

doubt then an ellipse biopsy should be taken through the most palpable part of the annular edge or a group of the most prominent papules in the generalized form.

Treatment is firstly reassurance as to the nature of the disease and the likelihood of spontaneous resolution. Where localized GA is disabling due to itch or disfigurement, then first-line treatment is with strong topical steroids, mometasone furoate or clobetasol diproprionate being suitable choices. These should be applied once daily to the advancing edge. Intralesional steroids injected into the advancing edge may be effective if topical steroids are not working but run a greater risk of steroid-induced atrophy and the procedure is painful. Where a biopsy has been taken, the disease can resolve and other inflammatory insults such as cryotherapy can produce a similar result; one study showed an 80 per cent success rate.[4] Cryotherapy is painful and can leave pale scars, so is not without potential side effects. For generalized GA, if treatment is needed it must be systemic and PUVA or other light treatment is probably the treatment of choice (see Section 10.14). Many other systemics have been reported as helpful and include dapsone, hydroxychloroquine, the retinoid drugs acitretin and isotretinoin, cyclosporin, chlorambucil and potassium iodide.

More recently interest has been generated by reports of the new topical T-cell specific inhibitor, tacrolimus, being effective in treatment of localized and generalized GA.[5,6] This treatment has the advantage of not producing atrophy and, if proven to be effective, would replace topical steroids as a treatment of choice. Imiquimod, the toll-like receptor 7 agonist that increases the innate immune response (licensed for treatment of genital warts and superficial skin cancers), has also shown some successes.[7] Finally, as yet unreported, the use of the thiazolidinediones has shown some good results in localized and generalized GA, interestingly in both diabetic and non-diabetic patients.

10.3 Necrobiosis Lipoidica

Necrobiosis lipoidica (Figure 10.5) typically presents as one or several red/brown asymptomatic papules or plaques on the anterior shins. Over a period of months these expand and the central area becomes atrophic with prominent telangiectasia and a yellow, xanthochromic appearance due to the underlying fat being visible through the thinned dermis. The overlying skin texture is shiny and often finely wrinkled to give an appearance similar to cigarette paper. Other sites can be involved, especially the feet and other areas on the lower leg, and involvement of the upper limbs, trunk and face can occur in up to 15 per cent of patients.[8] Approximately two-thirds of patient will have diabetes at onset and some of the remainder will go on to develop diabetes. Young adults are most commonly affected, although it is described at all ages, and it is more common in females. In the non-diabetic population the age of onset is later and up to 85 per cent are female. It does not seem to be related to the duration of diabetes nor to the effectiveness of glycaemic control. The disease is often long-standing and the plaques will continue to expand for some years before becoming "burnt out" when the advancing red/brown nodular edge disappears, leaving the central xanthochromic atrophy and macular brown post-inflammatory hyperpigmentation.

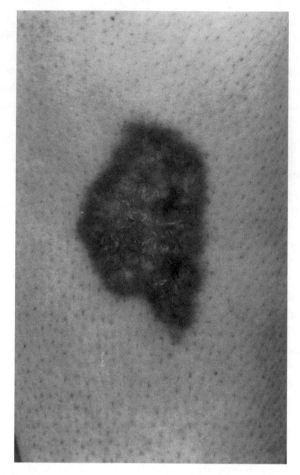

Figure 10.5 Typical necrobiosis lipoidica, here seen on the shin of a young diabetic girl

In the early stages the papules can be mistaken for granuloma annulare and other granulomatous disease such as sarcoidosis, but generally diagnosis is not difficult.

Unless ulcerated, treatment is cosmetic, but particularly as this affects a young population and can be the only visible stigmata of a patient's diabetes, distress can be considerable. Many treatments have been tried which, as usual, means that none are universally successful. Strong topical steroids can be applied to the area and then occluded overnight with a covering of clingfilm to aid penetration. If this is unsuccessful then injecting steroid into the advancing edge can help to suppress the disease, but as this is a disease with marked atrophy, the steroids, both injected and topical, can worsen this. The aim of this treatment is to settle the active disease and it is important for the patient to know that the atrophy will remain when making their decision as to whether to undergo treatment. Owing to a possible microvascular aetiology, several treatments concentrate on improving blood flow. A combination of aspirin and dipyridamole has been reported to be successful, although a trial of 300 mg aspirin and 75 mg dipyridamole showed no benefit.[9] Nicotinamide has shown benefit in reducing redness and pain in an open study;[10] although the benefits are probably small, the risk of side effects is minimal. Pentoxifylline[11] and intravenous prostaglandin have been reported as helpful, as has hyperbaric oxygen and hydroxychloroquine.[12] Successful treatment by excision and skin graft has been described, but recurrence can occur in the graft. The persistent telangiectasia can be treated with pulsed dye laser.[13] Once ulcerated

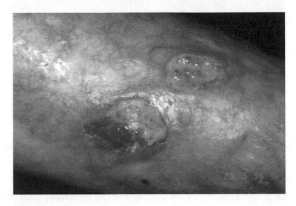

Figure 10.6   Ulcerated necrobiosis lipoidica (courtesy of Dr Richard Ashton, Haslar Hospital, Gosport)

(Figure 10.6), necrobiosis lipoidica becomes a much greater problem and potential health risk. If topical treatments are not helping, then oral steroids up to 60 mg of prednisolone daily or admitting the patient for pulsed intravenous steroids with methyl prednisolone is helpful despite the temporary worsening of their diabetic control. Topical PUVA[14] and cyclosporin[15,16] would be the next treatments to consider. Mycophenolate mofetil,[17] GM-CSF[18] and infliximab[19] have been reported as beneficial, as has engineered skin grafting.[20]

There are several reports of squamous cell carcinoma arising in necrobiosis lipoidica and so this complication should be considered in patients whose disease develops expansile nodules or where ulceration progresses with thickening at the periphery.[21,22]

10.4   Acanthosis Nigricans

Acanthosis nigricans (Figure 10.7) is a group of conditions that show pigmented, hyperkeratotic skin, usually in the flexures that are associated with hyperinsulinaemia. Medical students are forever on the lookout for the malignancy-associated acanthosis nigricans, but almost always it is associated with obesity and so is

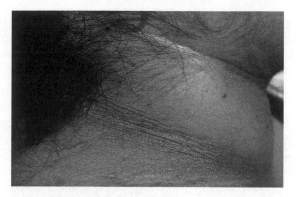

Figure 10.7   Acanthosis nigracans; typical hyperpigmented, velvety plaques occurring in the flexures in pigmented skin (courtesy of Dr Richard Ashton, Haslar Hospital, Gosport)

becoming more commonly seen in our affluent society. In all, six types are recognized. The most common is pseudoacanthosis nigricans, which occurs with obesity and hyperinsulinaemia. It shows a strong racial disposition to dark skins and so is common in Indian, Hispanic and black populations. The other five are the malignancy-associated form, a drug-induced, hereditary benign form, a very rare naevoid form and a benign form that is associated with other endocrinopathies such as HAIR-AN (hyperandrogenism, insulin resistance, acanthosis nigricans) syndrome.

The typical presentation is of warty, pigmented, poorly defined plaques that occur in the axillae, groin and neck and have a velvety feel to them due to being made up from multiple tiny papules. The neck changes have been described as 'dirty neck'. The onset is gradual, starting in childhood if weight is greater than 200 per cent of ideal and increasing at puberty. As the disease progresses and the plaques thicken further, the papules may become larger and form multiple skin tags, small 2–5 mm pedunculated, skin-coloured papules. The malignancy-associated variant usually shows a sudden onset of more severe disease. The palms are almost always affected – tripe palms – and the mucous membranes show similar warty hyperkeratosis. Many tumours have been linked, including those of bronchus, kidney, oesophagus and rectum. Associated suspicious symptoms, late, sudden onset, lack of obesity and involvement of palms or mucous membranes should initiate a search for neoplasia.

The condition is caused by hyperinsulinaemia. Keratinocytes possess insulin-like growth factor receptors which when stimulated increase DNA synthesis and cell proliferation. The most usual presentation in Portsmouth is in middle-aged obese Indians who already have or are developing type 2 diabetes. Treatment is by weight reduction, but vitamin D analogues[23] and oral[24,25] and topical[26] retinoids have been tried with success. Metformin seems to be effective.[25,27]

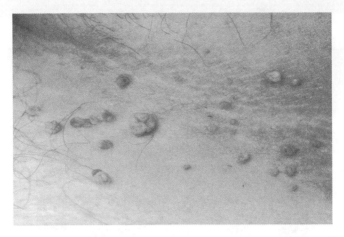

Figure 10.8 Acanthosis nigracans with multiple skin tags, here in Caucasian skin (courtesy of Dr Richard Ashton, Haslar Hospital, Gosport)

The thiazolidinediones certainly improve insulin resistance, but as yet have not been reported as directly improving acanthosis nigricans, although they would seem to be ideal for this use. The troublesome skin tags (Figure 10.8) can be removed by cryotherapy, shave excision or simple cautery, but since there may be several hundred, it is usually best to teach the patient or their spouse to make a loop in a length of cotton and drop this over the skin tag, lassoing it, and then pulling tight and knotting off. The tag will become inflamed and sore over a couple of days and then drop off. Even in diabetic patients there is minimal risk from this type of 'surgery'.

10.5   Eruptive Xanthomata

Eruptive xanthomata (Figure 10.9) is another of the typical medical student and MRCP candidate conditions, frequently looked for, seen in exams and rarely seen in the clinic. The case illustrated was presented to me in 2004. He was a 57-year-old man with type 2 diabetes of 10 years' duration. These multiple yellow papules had developed on his extensor surfaces over a 6 week period with slight itching. His triglyceride level was 37 mmol/l. Typically the papules are 1–2 mm in diameter with a red base and yellow domed top. They are usually itchy and may be associated with a triglyceride level of several thousand. Their importance is in recognizing this and the associated risk of pancreatitis. Lipaemia retinalis may also be present. Treatment is by improving glycaemic control and dietary fat reduction. Rewardingly, with treatment of the hypertriglyceridaemia, the papules will quickly disappear.

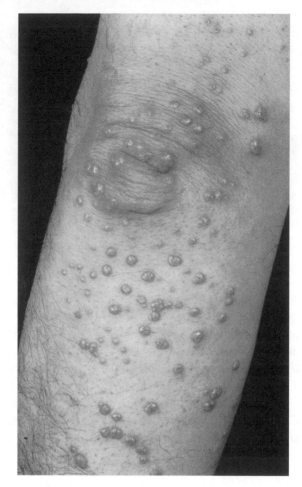

Figure 10.9 Eruptive xanthomata with multiple xanthochromic papules on the extensor surfaces and buttocks

10.6 Diabetic Thick Skin

In the skin diabetes simulates a premature ageing syndrome. Collagen's age can be determined by its resistance to enzymatic degradation and Hamlin *et al*[28] showed that young patients who had died of their diabetes had tendon collagen that degraded similarly to that of normal controls 60 years their senior. The glycosylation of collagen within the dermis and blood vessel endothelium underlies much of the pathology in this condition and in the skin produces a group of conditions that are described separately but really are part of a spectrum of disorders. Diabetic thick skin includes the conditions limited joint mobility, scleroderma-like syndrome and scleroedema diabeticorum.

Limited joint mobility

This condition is why all patients at diabetic review are asked to make a prayer sign. Thickening of the collagen within the skin and connective tissue around joints produces reduced mobility and thickened waxy skin. The little finger is the first affected and the disease progresses laterally to affect all digits. As the joint itself is uninvolved the synonym 'cheiroarthropathy,' is misleading. Detection is by the prayer sign where affected individuals are unable to oppose their palms when asked. The true importance of this condition is that it is closely related to retinopathy and nephropathy and is the earliest marker for these complications.[29-31] The use of this condition as a marker seems to decrease as patients become chronologically older, and is more significant in children and young patients with diabetes.[32] Thirty-five per cent of adolescent patients with insulin-dependant diabetes suffer from limited joint mobility,[33] more commonly in the subtalar joint than those of the hands. The proportion of non-insulin-dependent diabetics affected is reported to range from 10 to 85 per cent. Poor diabetic control is a risk factor for development of the condition, with a 46 per cent increased risk of the disease for every raised unit of Hba1C,[34] and tight control will gradually reduce the stiffness. Pleasingly, Infante *et al*[35] showed a fourfold reduction in the prevalence of limited joint mobility in children between 1976 and 1998, ascribing this to the improved glycaemic control over this period.

Scleroderma-like syndrome

Often associated with limited joint mobility, scleroderma-like syndrome presents with thickened waxy skin over the dorsa of the hands and feet. Around the knuckles there may be tiny papules. It is reported in 5–25 per cent of diabetic patients and is linked to the duration of the disease. Treatment is with improved glycaemic control.

Diabetic scleroedema

Scleroedema is a localized induration and thickening of the skin that can be either post-infective, associated with blood dyscrasias or associated with diabetes.[36] It should not be confused with the rather similar sounding condition scleroderma, which for us dyslexics has always been a difficult distinction. Onset is gradual and usually involves the neck, upper back and face. The face can become expressionless. Involvements of shoulders, upper limbs and trunk can then follow. Truncal and lower limb involvement is rare but reported. The skin develops a hard, woody, thickened feel. There may be restriction of movement of joints, and pharyngeal involvement with dysphagia has been reported. It is described as rare but this probably represents under-reporting, with one study finding the condition in 14 per cent of diabetic patients.[37] Scleroedema is most common in obese non-insulin diabetics who are often difficult to control and go on to need insulin; however, it is not associated with an increase risk in other diabetic complications, although this has not been universally found.[37] Investigation should include an ASO titre and a screen for a paraproteinaemia to exclude other causes of the scleroedema. Treatment has been attempted with methotrexate[38] and prostaglandin E_1,[39] but the most promising treatment is radiotherapy.[40–42]

10.7   Diabetic Dermopathy

Diabetic dermopathy (Figure 10.10) presents as asymptomatic pigmented, scaly papules and plaques on the shins, hence the alias 'shin spots'. It is common and occurs in 24 per cent of diabetic patients[43] and 40 per cent over 50 years.[44] Their

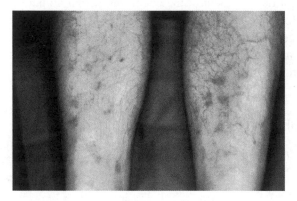

Figure 10.10   Diabetic dermopathy (courtesy of Dr Richard Ashton, Haslar Hospital, Gosport)

importance is their link to other diabetic complications such as retinopathy, neuropathy and nephropathy. They start as multiple small brown macules that develop fine scale and over a period of a few years will fade to leave subtle atrophic scars. At this stage they are difficult to see, but because they are continually being produced it seems to the patient as if they do not go away. They are thought to be related to microangiopathy and endothelial basement membrane thickening with glycosylated collagen, although a recent laser Doppler study demonstrated increased blood flow in the macules;[45] this does not, of course, exclude a prior vascular insult. They are more common as the duration of diabetes increases. Since their first naming in 1965[46] they have been described in normal individuals. Treatment is unnecessary as they will resolve on their own but moisturization may help if symptoms are troublesome.

10.8 Bullosis Diabeticorum

Bullosis diabeticorum is rare, 44 cases being reported between its first description in 1967[47] and 1985.[48] It is now likely that more cases go unreported and the real importance of awareness of this condition is to prevent erroneous treatments of other blistering disorders. The bullae are of sudden onset, almost universally on the feet, although bullae on the hands have been reported in one case;[48] typically they are several centimetres in diameter, although smaller vesicles have been reported. They are filled with clear yellow fluid and the base of the blister is quiet, i.e. there is no inflammation around the blister. An important diagnostic sign is that they are not itchy. They heal with no scarring over a few weeks. There is some support for them being fragility-based in that suction blisters can be produced more easily in diabetic skin.[49]

The main differential diagnosis is bullous pemphigoid, in which intensely itchy large bullae occur on the lower leg, arm and occasionally the trunk, of elderly patients (over 65 years) with surrounding erythema and urticaria. A biopsy should be taken for normal histology and a sample sent for immunofluorescence. This will demonstrate the immunobullous nature of pemphigoid with a band of IgG and C_3 demonstrable at the dermoepidermal junction. Routine histology in bullosis diabeticorum shows a blister split between the dermis and epidermis with very little reaction in the surrounding skin, hence the thick-walled tense blister in a quiet background. Bullous pemphigoid shows a split at a similar level, giving the same blister, but the surrounding skin shows an intense infiltrate with many eosinophils, which is clinically seen with an inflammatory base to the blisters and surrounding urticaria. Most laboratories can also demonstrate the relevant skin autoantibody on serum. As pemphigoid is much more common than bullosis diabeticorum and needs high-dose oral steroid treatment, differentiating these two conditions is vital. Porphyria cutanea tarda can present with blistering of the hands in a photo-exposed distribution and may be seen in a diabetic population due to the link with haemochromatosis, so porphyrins should be measured in patients with more prominent involvement on the upper limbs. Other causes of thick-walled tense blisters are drug-induced, e.g. barbiturates, and thermal or chemical burns. As the condition is self-limiting, no specific treatment is necessary.

10.9 Infections

Diabetic patients are at greater risk of certain infections and of increased severity.

Bacterial infections

Staphylococcal skin infections were previously a presenting feature of diabetes, but with more modern antibiotic use this has decreased. It is only over the last few years that a rise in methicillin-resistant *Staphylococcus aureus* (MRSA) has begun to be increasingly important in the diabetic group.[50] Streptococcal infections are increased in diabetic patients and one study showed a 30-fold increase risk for group B streptococcal infections,[51] and a significant mortality of up to 20 per cent, despite treatment. The most common sites of infection were cellulitis and foot and decubitus ulcers. The risk for group A streptococcal infections is less at 3.7 times.[52]

Malignant otitis externa is a infection of the external auditory meatus, usually caused by *Pseudomonas*, that is very invasive and can cause cranial osteomyelitis and intracranial involvement. Most patients have diabetes and mortality is between 20 and 40 per cent. Patients complain of painful, unilateral facial swelling and aural discharge and hearing loss.

Necrotizing fasciitis is also more common in diabetics with about two-thirds of diagnosed cases being diabetic. It is a polymicrobial infection, usually of the legs, perineum and abdomen with *E. coli*, *Bacteroides* and *Clostridium* being commonly involved. The infection spreads along fascial planes and the patient presents with induration, erythema, necrosis and bullae formation. Pain is often severe and the patient is more toxic than would be expected from the clinical signs. Surgical debridement and appropriate antibiotics are urgently needed.

Fungal infections

Candida infections are more common in diabetes including intertrigo, genital, oral and nail infections. Dermatophyte infections are also more common, with toenail onychomycosis nearly three times more common in diabetic patients. Given the risk of cellulitis in this group, it is important to treat this potential portal of infection. Topical treatment can be effective but oral terbinafine, despite rare hepatitis, has a risk–benefit ratio that is heavily in favour of treatment. Three months of treatment are necessary to treat a toenail infection adequately.

A rare severe infection by the opportunistic fungus *Zygomycetes* is rhinocerebral mucormycosis. This presents with nasal swelling and pain associated with headache and lethargy. Most patients with this condition have diabetes and mortality is up to 30 per cent. Treatment is with surgical debridement and amphotericin B.

10.10   Perforating Disorders

This is an interesting group of disorders in which dermal components such as collagen and elastin are extruded through the epidermis, so-called 'transepidermal elimination'. This can be secondary to other dermatoses, for instance perforating granuloma annulare, but four primary dermatological variants are recognized: Kyrle's disease, perforating folliculitis, reactive perforating collagenosis and perforating serpiginous elastosis. Each is a distinct entity divided by its appearance, what is extruded, response to trauma and clinical characteristics; however, all can be seen in diabetics and renal failure. They are particularly common during dialysis,[53,54] occurring in up to 10 per cent of patients. A new diagnosis of acquired reactive perforating dermatosis was suggested to cover this group.[55] When originally described, these conditions were thought to be related to scratching[56] and there is still some evidence to support this;[57] however, damage to collagen and accumulation of 'uraemic substances' have also been postulated. Clinically the patients present with itchy papules on the limbs and trunk with a keratotic centre. These grow over a few weeks to several millimetres in diameter, rarely a centimetre, and then settle to leave hypopigmentation and some slight scarring. In patients suspected of this disorder, first a biopsy should be taken that includes one complete, fresh papule that is not too excoriated. This shows the altered collagen being extruded within a cup of thickened epidermis surrounded by a mild lymphocytic infiltrate. Alerting the pathologist to the clinical diagnosis will allow them arrange special stains for collagen which are very useful. Renal function should be checked and also other causes of pruritus looked for: iron deficiency and anaemia, liver enzyme abnormalities and thyroid abnormalities. Treatment is not universally successful and patients often continue to develop papules. Strong topical steroids have been reported as useful,[58] as have topical retinoids,[59] UVB[60] and PUVA,[58] TENS[61] for itching and allopurinol.[62,63]

10.11 Glucagonoma Syndrome

This is a very rare syndrome with the presence of a glucagonoma and hyperglucagonaemia characterized by diabetes or abnormal glucose tolerance, weight loss and a characteristic rash, necrolytic migratory erythema. It may occur as part of a multiple endocrine neoplasia syndrome. The patient is usually in the sixth to eighth decade and presents with non-specific symptoms of malaise, weight loss, diabetes and stomatitis. The rash is an itchy and painful eruption that mainly involves the flexures, particularly the groin, starting with an erythematous patch that blisters and then expands to form annular and arcuate plaques. The central area heals with pigmentation and then tends to recur over a period of 10 days. The eruption can be very subtle and diagnosis can be delayed, sometimes for years. At presentation 50 per cent of patients will have metastatic disease. The cause of the rash is unknown, but it is similar to that seen in acrodermatitis enteropathica, which is related to low zinc levels. Necrolytic migratory erythema has been described as resolving with zinc and amino acid supplementation as well as with resection of the tumour. Diagnosis is clinical as, although the pathological changes are very suggestive, they can be subtle and easily missed. A biopsy should be taken from the blistering area or advancing active edge. This will show a lymphohistiocytic infiltrate with eosinophils and neutrophils, but with a characteristic split in the epidermis with a necrotic overlying layer. Not all cases of necrolytic migratory erythema are associated with a glucagonoma and may be seen in cirrhosis (reduced metabolism of glucagon), coelic disease and cystic fibrosis. Further investigation should include glucagon, insulin, gastrin and VIP levels. Zinc, amino acid and essential fatty acid levels should be checked for possible therapeutic supplementation. Radiology to define the tumour and any metastatic disease should include CT, MRI and coeliac axis angiography. Treatment is by surgical excision.

10.12 Vitiligo

Not a true diabetic complication, vitiligo (Figure 10.11) is seen in association with several autoimmune endocrine diseases and so is included here. These diseases are

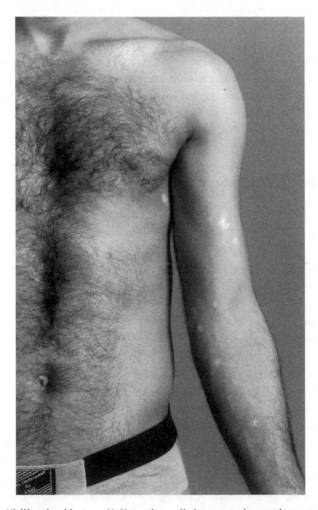

Figure 10.11 Vitiligo in skin type V. Note the well-demarcated non-pigmented patches

hyper- and hypothyroidism, Addison's disease, diabetes and hypoparathyroidism. It is also seen in conjunction with pernicious anaemia and myasthenia gravis. It common in the general population with prevalence estimated at 1 per cent and, when seen in children, it is most likely to be in association with other disorders. It is more common in pigmented skin and has a much higher social morbidity in darker skins, particularly in Indians, due to the link of hypopigmented patches with leprosy. Vitiligo is not hypopigmented, but amelanotic, i.e. it is not pale skin but completely depigmented. It tends to be symmetrical and occurs on photo-exposed sites and those susceptible to trauma. It koebenerizes (occurs in trauma and scars). Differential diagnosis includes post-inflammatory hypopigmentation. This can follow any inflammatory skin disease, particularly in darker skins, but a previous inflammatory phase is usually evident, often with the presence of itching. Vitiligo is asymptomatic, although it will be painful after sunburn. Leprosy can be diagnosed by the presence of anaesthesia to light touch in the patches and palpable thickened nerves, best felt over the elbow. Other hypopigmented dermatoses can be excluded by the use of a Wood's lamp. This ultraviolet lamp when used to view the patient in a darkened room will highlight the areas of pigmentary change and can be used to show the variable pigment levels in other dermatoses. These should not be present in vitiligo. Autoantibodies can be demonstrated directed against melanocytes, but those in hair follicles seem to be spared. The condition is self-limiting in 20–30 per cent of patients and, particularly after ultraviolet exposure, one may see spotty repigmentation as melanocytes migrate out of uninvolved hair follicles. Treatment depends on the extent of the disease, disability and skin type. Caucasian skin is difficult to treat and thus reassurance and cosmetic camouflage are used. As the skin type darkens, so the chance of therapeutic benefit increases. Traditionally PUVA was the treatment of choice (Figure 10.12), but successful results have been shown with vitamin D analogues, topical retinoids and, most promisingly, tacrolimus. Multiple other treatments have been used, including many different ultraviolet regimes, excimer laser and melanocyte culture and reimplantation, none being universally helpful. It is important to adequately protect the patches from the sun, as they will burn easily. A suitable treatment protocol would be: for Caucasian skin – reassure, cosmetic camouflage and tacrolimus; for type V/VI skin – consider referral for PUVA.

10.13   Dermatological Definitions

Dermatologists speak a different language. Like Eskimos and snow, we need 100 words for 'spots' and 50 words for 'red'. It has been shown that we do have increased sensitivity in discerning levels of redness and we have even tried to develop machines to do this for us – erythema meters. As our clinical meetings often illustrate, show 10 dermatologists a rash and they will describe it in 10 different ways, suggest 10 different diagnoses but, as our critics say, still treat it

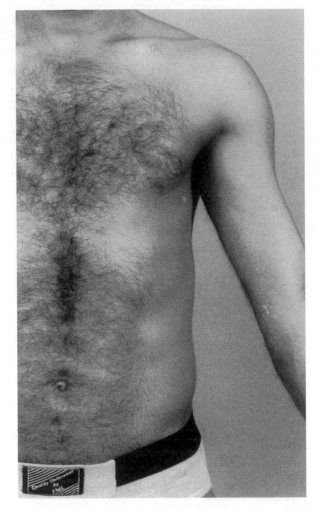

Figure 10.12   Figure 10.11 after 10 weeks of PUVA treatment. Note partial repigmentation

with topical steroids. There are, however, some constants in our vocabulary and
below is a list of terms that I have used in this chapter:

- papules – raised area less than 5 mm in diameter;

- plaques – a flat-topped raised area greater than 5 mm in diameter;

- pedunculated – a papule with a narrow neck where it joins the skin;

- macules – an area of altered colour or texture that is not raised and generally
  less than 1 cm in diameter;

- patch – a flat coloured area larger than 1 cm;

- vesicle – a blister less than 5 mm in diameter;

- bulla – a blister greater than 5 mm in diameter;

- ulcer – an area of skin that has lost the epidermal layer;

- hyperkeratosis – thickening of the skin due to accumulation of keratin;

- telangiectasia – dilation of small blood vessels visible to the naked eye;

- erythema – redness of the skin due to vasodilation;

- pigmentation – brown discolouration of skin that can be either due to melanin from melanocytes or haemosiderin (digested blood leaking from blood vessels);

- violaceous – purple discolouration of skin;

- xanthochromia – yellow discolouration of skin;

- annular – in a ring;

- linear – in a line.

10.14 Dermatological Therapeutics

For non-dermatologists one of the most confusing areas is dermatological treatment. We use a very different armamentarium of therapies from creams and ointments to destructive therapies and ultraviolet radiation. This section details short notes on these therapies so that the reader can explain to their patient the likely types of treatment available and the risks.

Topical treatments

These come in either cream or ointment form. Ointments are in a Vaseline (petrolatum) base and are thick and greasy. They are preferred by dermatologists since they have a significant moisturizing effect as well as the effect from any other active ingredients. They contain no preservatives. Creams are milky and often preferred by patients as they massage into the skin more easily. They have a higher concentration of water than ointments and so may be a reservoir for bacteria, thus they need preservatives that are a potential cause of sensitization and allergic contact dermatitis. If in doubt, prescribe an ointment and only use a cream where the alternative is cosmetically unacceptable to the patient or on hairy areas or mucous membranes.

Topical steroids are useful for treating granuloma annulare, necrobiosis lipoidica and perforating disorders. They come in four potencies. It is prudent to know one or two examples from each potency. Mild steroids include hydrocortisone and can be applied without risk of side effects such as skin thinning. They are safe for long-term use on the face and available over the counter in the UK. Moderate potency steroids would include clobetasone butyrate (Eumovate). They are safe for long-term use on the body and short term on the face (1–2 weeks). Examples of potent topical steroids are betamethasone valerate (Betnovate) or mometasone furoate (Elocon), which can be used short-term on the body, they should be avoided on the face except under expert supervision and should be used with extreme care in the flexures. Clobetasol propionate (Dermovate) is a very potent topical steroid and should be used with care. In conditions such as granuloma annulare and necrobiosis lipoidica it can be used under clingfilm occlusion to increase its penetration. There is a severe risk of atrophy with this if it is not undertaken correctly.

All steroid creams should be applied daily. Although some creams suggest twice daily dosing there is no good evidence that this is necessary and a five-days-out-of-seven regime may help to present tachyphylaxis. In Portsmouth all patients are advised to use their topical steroids in the evening Monday to Friday and restrict themselves to moisturizing creams at the weekend. Side effects are usually related to the potency of the cream. Skin atrophy and striae are those most feared by patients but in fact are rarely seen nowadays. Cutaneous infections, particularly staphylococcal, can be worsened by treatment with topical steroids, but the addition of either a topical or oral antibiotic will be adequate where the steroid treatment needs to be continued. Cataracts have been reported with long-term use of potent or very potent creams on the eyelids, but not with mild alternatives. They may precipitate acne or perioral dermatitis (multiple papules, pustules and vesicles occurring around the mouth with a clear border around the lips) and should then be discontinued.

Vitamin D analogues are most commonly prescribed for psoriasis but have been used in treatment of acanthosis nigricans. Calcipotriol (Dovonex), calcitriol (Silkis) and tacalcitol (Curatoderm) are the three products available. They bind to the steroid family of nuclear super receptors and reduce cell turnover and therefore hyperkeratosis. Side effects are usually local with redness and irritation being the most common. Overuse can theoretically cause hypercalcaemia and care should be taken in renal failure or dysfunction. Calcipotriol should be limited to 100 g per week and calcitriol to less than 35 per cent of body surface area, but neither of these is likely to be reached in treating acanthosis nigricans.

Topical retinoids are useful for treating the perforating disorders and acanthosis nigricans and are supplied in cream or gel form. They are vitamin A derivatives and can be quite difficult for the patient to use as they can irritate the skin. Adapalene is probably the least irritant and I would recommend the 0.1 per cent cream (Differin cream) where it is needed. They should be applied initially once daily and then, after 1 week if irritation does not occur, twice daily. They can make the skin more susceptible to sunburn and so ultraviolet avoidance or good sun protection may be needed.

Tacrolimus is a topical immunomodulator that is a cyclosporin analogue, however, unlike cyclosporin, it is active topically as it is a smaller molecule and able to penetrate the skin. It has been used to treat both granuloma annulare and necrobiosis lipoidica and works by suppressing antigen-specific T-cell activation and inhibiting inflammatory cytokine release. It acts similarly to a topical steroid but does not have the skin-thinning side effects. It is an ointment that is used twice daily and patients must be warned that it is likely to sting for the first few applications. This is due to local release of substance P from nerve endings that are then depleted of this chemical, allowing the side effect to subside. Other side effects include worsening or precipitation of skin infections, particularly *Herpes simplex*, and some patient flush if they concurrently drink alcohol. There is a theoretical risk that the reduction in skin immune surveillance could increase skin cancer risk and so ultraviolet light exposure should be minimized.

Imiquimod is licensed for the treatment of genital warts and superficial skin cancers but has also been used for treating granuloma annulare. It is a toll-like receptor 7 analogue that increases interferon-α, tumour necrosis factor and interleukin-12. It is applied from a sachet, usually three times per week, and causes a localized inflammatory reaction.

Cryotherapy

Cryotherapy is the application of liquid nitrogen to the skin to cause a controlled burn. It can be used to treat granuloma annulare and necrobiosis lipoidica. The liquid is sprayed on with a gun; the required area is frozen to achieve an ice ball and then maintained at that temperature for the given time, usually 10–30 s. It is painful and will often produce blistering followed by an eschar. This settles to leave some element of scaring and often post-inflammatory hypopigmentation.

Ultraviolet treatments

There are three types of ultraviolet treatment, broadband UVB, narrowband UVB and PUVA. They are listed in order of increasing efficacy but also of increasing potential side effects. In all cases the patient stands in an ultraviolet cabinet with the relevant area exposed. Face shields, clothes or sun block can protect areas not to be treated. The first treatments are often only for 10–15 s, but over a period of

10 weeks they can build up to 5–10 min exposure. The exposure time depends on a patient's skin type, and six test doses are shone onto the patient's arm to gauge the starting time. Ten weeks is the average course necessary for treatment.

UVB is given three times weekly and so the patient must be able to attend the department this frequently and also be able to stand in the cabinet for the necessary exposure. Elderly and infirm patients may be treated supine if a suitable machine is available. Children often tolerate the procedure well and a parent can sit by the cabinet in their line of sight to give moral support. Side effects are mainly the risk of burning. Narrow-band UVB is a newer modality where the ultraviolet rays are concentrated around 311 nm. This seems to be more effective than broadband UVB, which uses a wide mix of wavelengths in the UVB spectrum. It has been shown to be as effective as PUVA in the treatment of psoriasis and has fewer side effects.

PUVA is the combination of a photosensitizer (Psoralens) and UVA. It can be given in three ways, topical, bath or oral, and is a twice-per-week regime, which may be easier for some patients. With topical PUVA a gel, Psoralens, is applied to a limited area, in bath treatment the patient lies in a bath with the Psoralens in the water for 15 min and in oral treatment they take a Psoralens tablet 2 h before treatment. The skin becomes sensitive to UVA and they are then exposed in a similar way to the UVB regime. Side effects are more common, including irritation and burning, photosensitivity of the treated area for 24 h (including the lens of the eye with oral PUVA), nausea with the oral regime and in all modalities, a definite increase risk in squamous cell carcinoma if more that 250 treatments are undertaken.

References

1. Nebesio CL, Lewis C, Chuang TY. Lack of an association between granuloma annulare and type 2 diabetes mellitus. *Br J Dermatol* 2002; **146**(1): 122–124.
2. Muhlemann MF, Williams DR. Localized granuloma annulare is associated with insulin-dependent diabetes mellitus. *Br J Dermatol* 1984; **111**(3): 325–329.
3. Dabski K, Winkelmann RK. Generalized granuloma annulare: clinical and laboratory findings in 100 patients. *J Am Acad Dermatol* 1989; **20**(1): 39–47.
4. Blume-Peytavi U, Zouboulis CC, Jacobi H, Scholz A, Bisson S, Orfanos CE. Successful outcome of cryosurgery in patients with granuloma annulare. *Br J Dermatol* 1994; **130**(4): 494–497.
5. Jain S, Stephens CJ. Successful treatment of disseminated granuloma annulare with topical tacrolimus. *Br J Dermatol* 2004; **150**(5): 1042–1043.
6. Harth W, Linse R. Topical tacrolimus in granuloma annulare and necrobiosis lipoidica. *Br J Dermatol* 2004; **150**(4): 792–794.
7. Kuwahara RT, Naylor MF, Skinner RB. Treatment of granuloma annulare with topical 5% imiquimod cream. *Pediatr Dermatol* 2003; **20**(1): 90.
8. Kavanagh GM, Novelli M, Hartog M, Kennedy CT. Necrobiosis lipoidica – involvement of atypical sites. *Clin Exp Dermatol* 1993; **18**(6): 543–544.

9. Statham B, Finlay AY, Marks R. A randomized double blind comparison of an aspirin dipyridamole combination versus a placebo in the treatment of necrobiosis lipoidica. *Acta Dermatol Venereol* 1981; **61**(3): 270–271.

10. Handfield-Jones S, Jones S, Peachey R. High dose nicotinamide in the treatment of necrobiosis lipoidica. *Br J Dermatol* 1988; **118**(5): 693–696.

11. Basaria S, Braga-Basaria M. Necrobiosis lipoidica diabeticorum: response to pentoxiphylline. *J Endocrinol Invest* 2003; **26**(10): 1037–1040.

12. Nguyen K, Washenik K, Shupack J. Necrobiosis lipoidica diabeticorum treated with chloroquine. *J Am Acad Dermatol* 2002; **46**(2 Suppl Case Reports): S34–36.

13. Currie CL, Monk BE. Pulsed dye laser treatment of necrobiosis lipoidica: report of a case. *J Cutan Laser Ther* 1999; **1**(4): 239–241.

14. De Rie MA, Sommer A, Hoekzema R, Neumann HA. Treatment of necrobiosis lipoidica with topical psoralen plus ultraviolet A. *Br J Dermatol* 2002; **147**(4): 743–747.

15. Stanway A, Rademaker M, Newman P. Healing of severe ulcerative necrobiosis lipoidica with cyclosporin. *Australas J Dermatol* 2004; **45**(2): 119–122.

16. Stinco G, Parlangeli ME, De Francesco V, Frattasio A, Germino M, Patrone P. Ulcerated necrobiosis lipoidica treated with cyclosporin A. *Acta Dermatol Venereol* 2003; **83**(2): 151–153.

17. Reinhard G, Lohmann F, Uerlich M, Bauer R, Bieber T. Successful treatment of ulcerated necrobiosis lipoidica with mycophenolate mofetil. *Acta Dermatol Venereol* 2000; **80**(4): 312–313.

18. Evans AV, Atherton DJ. Recalcitrant ulcers in necrobiosis lipoidica diabeticorum healed by topical granulocyte-macrophage colony-stimulating factor. *Br J Dermatol* 2002; **147**(5): 1023–1025.

19. Kolde G, Muche JM, Schulze P, Fischer P, Lichey J. Infliximab: a promising new treatment option for ulcerated necrobiosis lipoidica. *Dermatology* 2003; **206**(2): 180–181.

20. Owen CM, Murphy H, Yates VM. Tissue-engineered dermal skin grafting in the treatment of ulcerated necrobiosis lipoidica. *Clin Exp Dermatol* 2001; **26**(2): 176–178.

21. Imtiaz KE, Khaleeli AA. Squamous cell carcinoma developing in necrobiosis lipoidica. *Diabet Med* 2001; **18**(4): 325–328.

22. Santos-Juanes J, Galache C, Curto JR, Carrasco MP, Ribas A, Sanchez del Rio J. Squamous cell carcinoma arising in long-standing necrobiosis lipoidica. *J Eur Acad Dermatol Venereol* 2004; **18**(2): 199–200.

23. Bohm M, Luger TA, Metze D. Treatment of mixed type acanthosis nigricans with topical calcipotriol. *Br J Dermatol* 1998; **139**(5): 932–934.

24. Akovbyan VA, Talanin NY, Arifov SS, Tukhvatullina ZG, Musabayev AN, Baybekov IM, Kang MK. Successful treatment of acanthosis nigricans with etretinate. *J Am Acad Dermatol* 1994; **31**(1): 118–120.

25. Walling HW, Messingham M, Myers LM, Mason CL, Strauss JS. Improvement of acanthosis nigricans on isotretinoin and metformin. *J Drugs Dermatol* 2003; **2**(6): 677–681.

26. Blobstein SH. Topical therapy with tretinoin and ammonium lactate for acanthosis nigricans associated with obesity. *Cutis* 2003; **71**(1): 33–34.

27. Tankova T, Koev D, Dakovska L, Kirilov G. Therapeutic approach in insulin resistance with acanthosis nigricans. *Int J Clin Pract* 2002; **56**(8): 578–581.

28. Hamlin CR, Kohn RR, Luschin JH. Apparent accelerated aging of human collagen in diabetes mellitus. *Diabetes* 1975; **24**(10): 902–904.

29. Rosenbloom AL, Silverstein JH, Lezotte DC, Richardson K, McCallum M. Limited joint mobility in childhood diabetes mellitus indicates increased risk for microvascular disease. *New Engl J Med* 1981; **305**(4): 191–194.

30. Garg SK, Chase HP, Marshall G, Jackson WE, Holmes D, Hoops S, Harris S. Limited joint mobility in subjects with insulin dependent diabetes mellitus: relationship with eye and kidney complications. *Arch Dis Child* 1992; **67**(1): 96–99.

31. Montana E, Rozadilla A, Nolla JM, Gomez N, Escofet DR, Soler J. Microalbuminuria is associated with limited joint mobility in type I diabetes mellitus. *Ann Rheum Dis* 1995; **54**(7): 582–586.

32. Haitas B, Jones DB, Ting A, Turner RC. Diabetic retinopathy and its association with limited joint mobility. *Horm Metab Res* 1986; **18**(11): 765–767.

33. Duffin AC, Donaghue KC, Potter M, McInnes A, Chan AK, King J, Howard NJ, Silink M. Limited joint mobility in the hands and feet of adolescents with type 1 diabetes mellitus. *Diabet Med* 1999; **16**(2): 125–130.

34. Silverstein JH, Gordon G, Pollock BH, Rosenbloom AL. Long-term glycemic control influences the onset of limited joint mobility in type 1 diabetes. *J Pediatr* 1998; **132**(6): 944–947.

35. Infante JR, Rosenbloom AL, Silverstein JH, Garzarella L, Pollock BH. Changes in frequency and severity of limited joint mobility in children with type 1 diabetes mellitus between 1976–78 and 1998. *J Pediatr* 2001; **138**(1): 33–37.

36. Fleischmajer R, Faludi G, Krol S. Scleredema and diabetes mellitus. *Arch Dermatol* 1970; **101**(1): 21–26.

37. Sattar MA, Diab S, Sugathan TN, Sivanandasingham P, Fenech FF. Scleroedema diabeticorum: a minor but often unrecognized complication of diabetes mellitus. *Diabet Med* 1988; **5**(5): 465–468.

38. Seyger MM, van den Hoogen FH, de Mare S, van Haelst U, de Jong EM. A patient with a severe scleroedema diabeticorum, partially responding to low-dose methotrexate. *Dermatology* 1999; **198**(2): 177–179.

39. Ikeda Y, Suehiro T, Abe T, Yoshida T, Shinoki T, Tahara K, Nishiyama M, Okabayashi T, Nakamura T, Itoh H, Hashimoto K. Severe diabetic scleredema with extension to the extremities and effective treatment using prostaglandin E1. *Intern Med* 1998; **37**(10): 861–864.

40. Konemann S, Hesselmann S, Bolling T, Grabbe S, Schuck A, Moustakis C, De Simoni D, Willich N, Micke O. Radiotherapy of benign diseases – scleredema adultorum Buschke. *Strahlenther Onkol* 2004; **180**(12): 811–814.

41. Bowen AR, Smith L, Zone JJ. Scleredema adultorum of Buschke treated with radiation. *Arch Dermatol* 2003; **139**(6): 780–784.

42. Tobler M, Leavitt DD, Gibbs FA Jr. Dosimetric evaluation of a specialized radiotherapy treatment technique for scleredema. *Med Dosim* 2000; **25**(4): 215–218.

43. Diris N, Colomb M, Leymarie F, Durlach V, Caron J, Bernard P. Non infectious skin conditions associated with diabetes mellitus: a prospective study of 308 cases. *Ann Dermatol Venereol* 2003; **130**(11): 1009–1014.

44. Shemer A, Bergman R, Linn S, Kantor Y, Friedman-Birnbaum R. Diabetic dermopathy and internal complications in diabetes mellitus. *Int J Dermatol* 1998; **37**(2): 113–115.

45. Wigington G, Ngo B, Rendell M. Skin blood flow in diabetic dermopathy. *Arch Dermatol* 2004; **140**(10): 1248–1250.

46. Binkley GW. Dermopathy in the diabetic syndrome. *Arch Dermatol* 1965; **92**(6): 625–634.

47. Cantwell AR Jr, Martz W. Idiopathic bullae in diabetics. Bullosis diabeticorum. *Arch Dermatol* 1967; **96**(1): 42–44.

48. Toonstra J. Bullosis diabeticorum. Report of a case with a review of the literature. *J Am Acad Dermatol* 1985; **13**(5 Pt 1): 799–805.

49. Bernstein JE, Levine LE, Medenica MM, Yung CW, Soltani K. Reduced threshold to suction-induced blister formation in insulin-dependent diabetics. *J Am Acad Dermatol* 1983; **8**(6): 790–791.

50. Dang CN, Prasad YD, Boulton AJ, Jude EB. Methicillin-resistant *Staphylococcus aureus* in the diabetic foot clinic: a worsening problem. *Diabet Med* 2003; **20**(2): 159–161.

51. Farley MM, Harvey RC, Stull T, Smith JD, Schuchat A, Wenger JD, Stephens DS. A population-based assessment of invasive disease due to group B *Streptococcus* in nonpregnant adults. *New Engl J Med* 1993; **328**(25): 1807–1811.

52. Davies HD, McGeer A, Schwartz B, Green K, Cann D, Simor AE, Low DE. Invasive group A streptococcal infections in Ontario, Canada. Ontario Group A Streptococcal Study Group. *New Engl J Med* 1996; **335**(8): 547–554.

53. Hurwitz RM, Melton ME, Creech FT 3rd, Weiss J, Handt A. Perforating folliculitis in association with hemodialysis. *Am J Dermatopathol* 1982; **4**(2): 101–108.

54. Morton CA, Henderson IS, Jones MC, Lowe JG. Acquired perforating dermatosis in a British dialysis population. *Br J Dermatol* 1996; **135**(5): 671–677.

55. Rapini RP, Herbert AA, Drucker CR. Acquired perforating dermatosis. Evidence for combined transepidermal elimination of both collagen and elastic fibers. *Arch Dermatol* 1989; **125**(8): 1074–1078.

56. Cochran RJ, Tucker SB, Wilkin JK. Reactive perforating collagenosis of diabetes mellitus and renal failure. *Cutis* 1983; **31**(1): 55–58.

57. Hong SB, Park JH, Ihm CG, Kim NI. Acquired perforating dermatosis in patients with chronic renal failure and diabetes mellitus. *J Korean Med Sci* 2004; **19**(2): 283–288.

58. Satchell AC, Crotty K, Lee S. Reactive perforating collagenosis: a condition that may be underdiagnosed. *Australas J Dermatol* 2001; **42**(4): 284–287.

59. Berger RS. Reactive perforating collagenosis of renal failure/diabetes responsive to topical retinoic acid. *Cutis* 1989; **43**(6): 540–542.

60. Ohe S, Danno K, Sasaki H, Isei T, Okamoto H, Horio T. Treatment of acquired perforating dermatosis with narrowband ultraviolet B. *J Am Acad Dermatol* 2004; **50**(6): 892–894.

61. Chan LY, Tang WY, Lo KK. Treatment of pruritis of reactive perforating collagenosis using transcutaneous electrical nerve stimulation. *Eur J Dermatol* 2000; **10**(1): 59–61.

62. Kruger K, Tebbe B, Krengel S, Goerdt S, Orfanos CE. Acquired reactive perforating dermatosis. Successful treatment with allopurinol in 2 cases. *Hautarzt* 1999; **50**(2): 115–120.

63. Munch M, Balslev E, Jemec GB. Treatment of perforating collagenosis of diabetes and renal failure with allopurinol. *Clin Exp Dermatol* 2000; **25**(8): 615–616.

Index

Figures and Tables are indicated by *italic page numbers*

Diabetes: Chronic Complications   Edited by Kenneth M. Shaw and Michael H. Cummings
© 2005 John Wiley & Sons, Ltd.